Cats

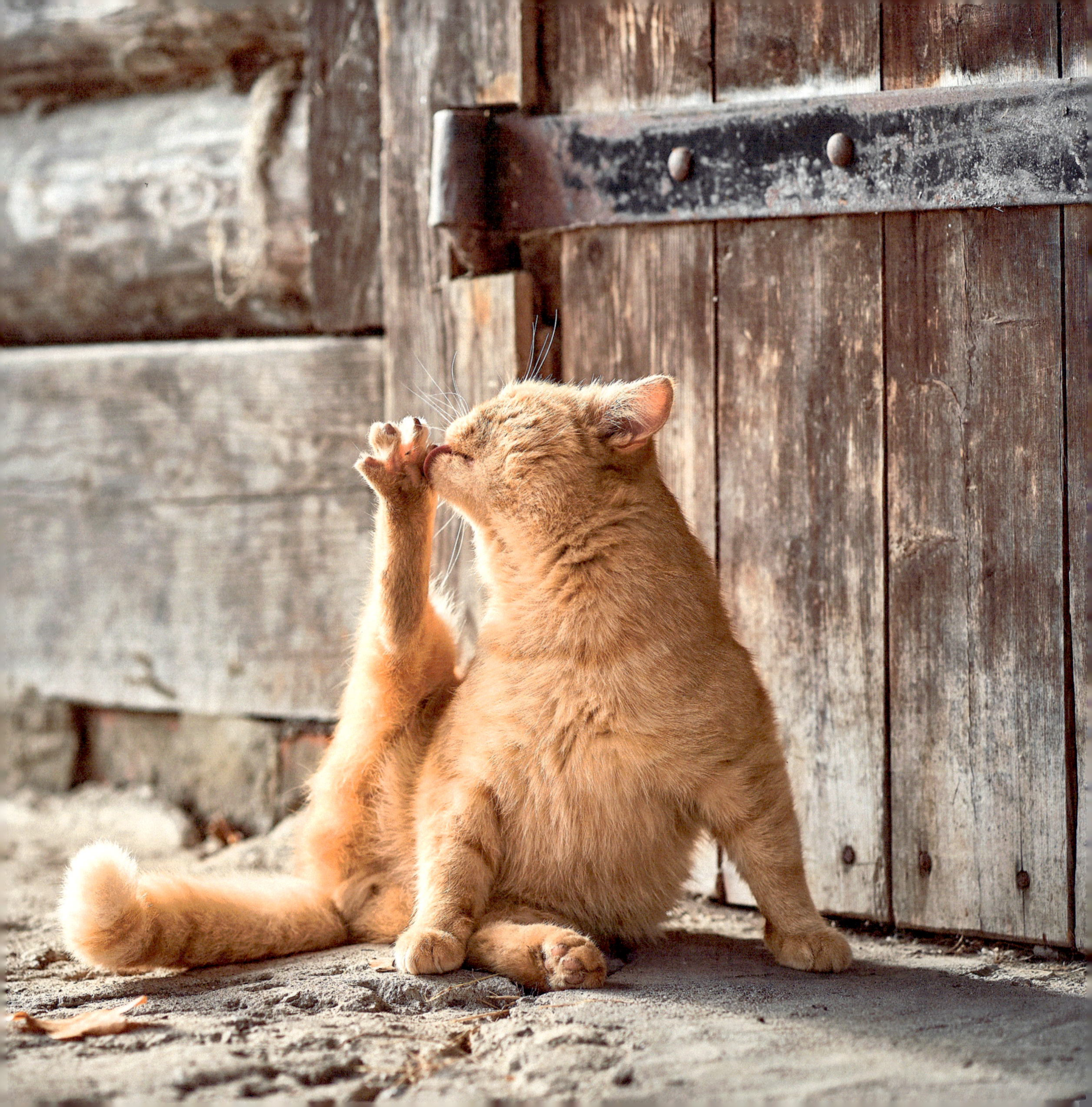

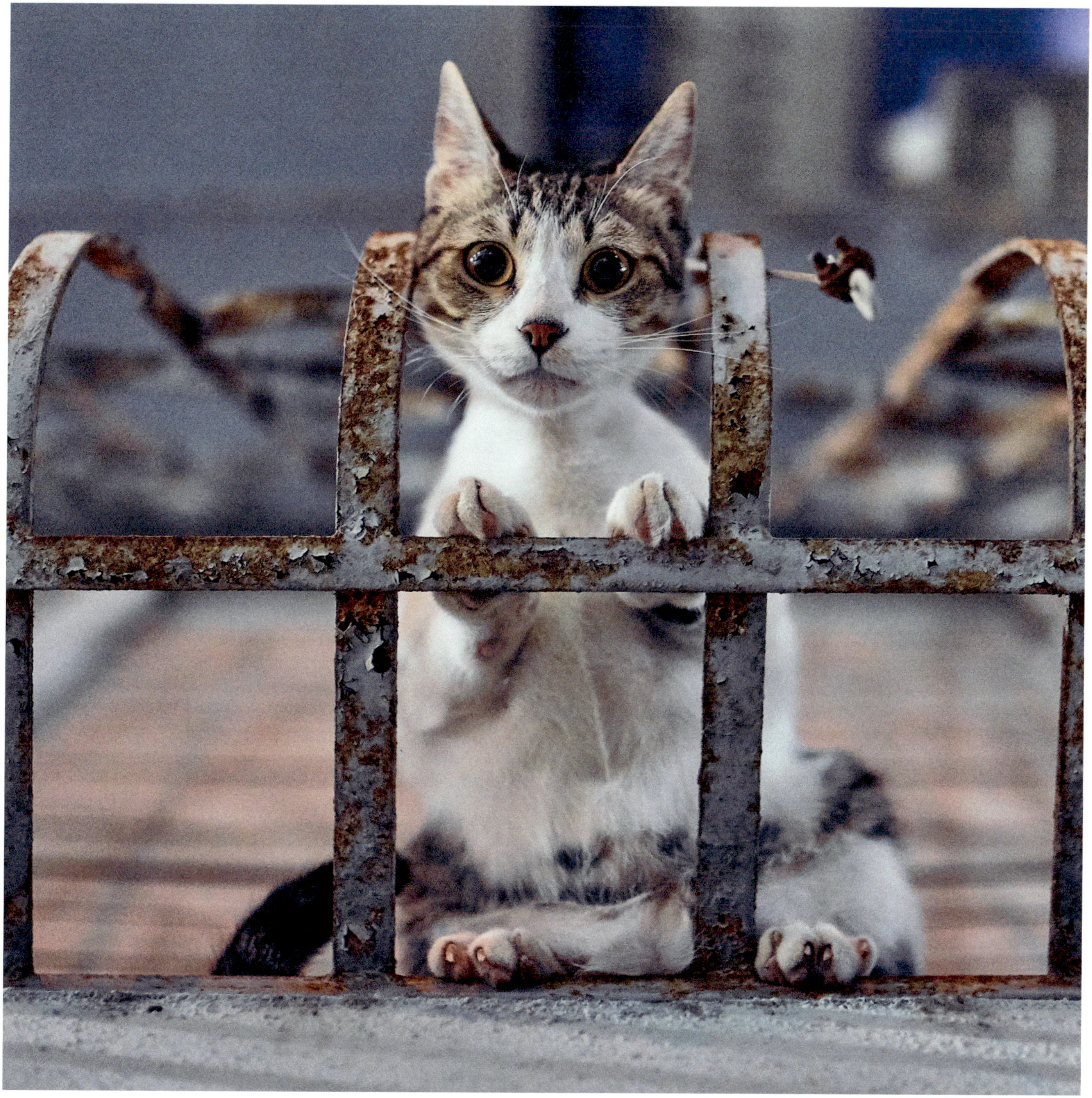

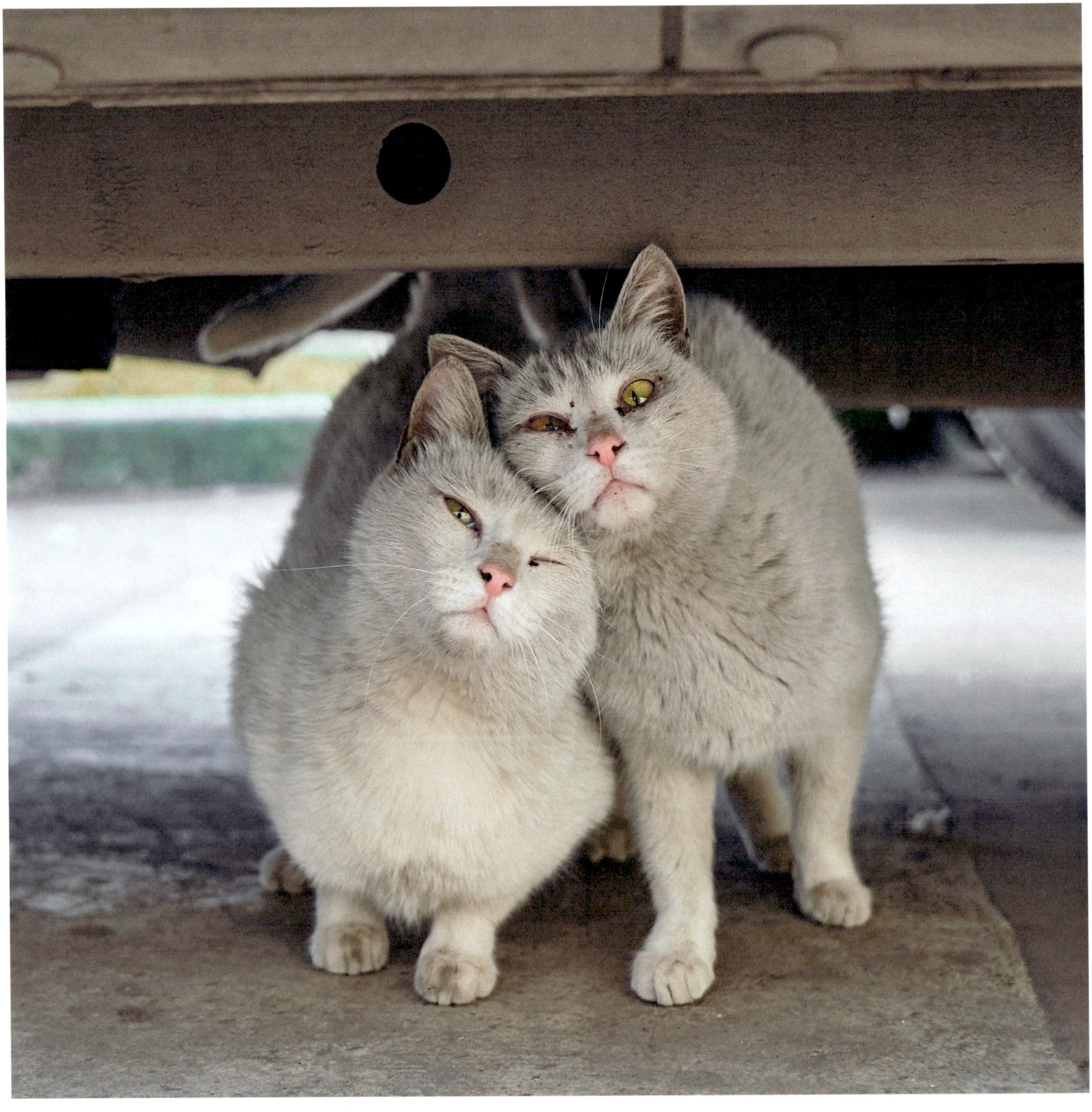

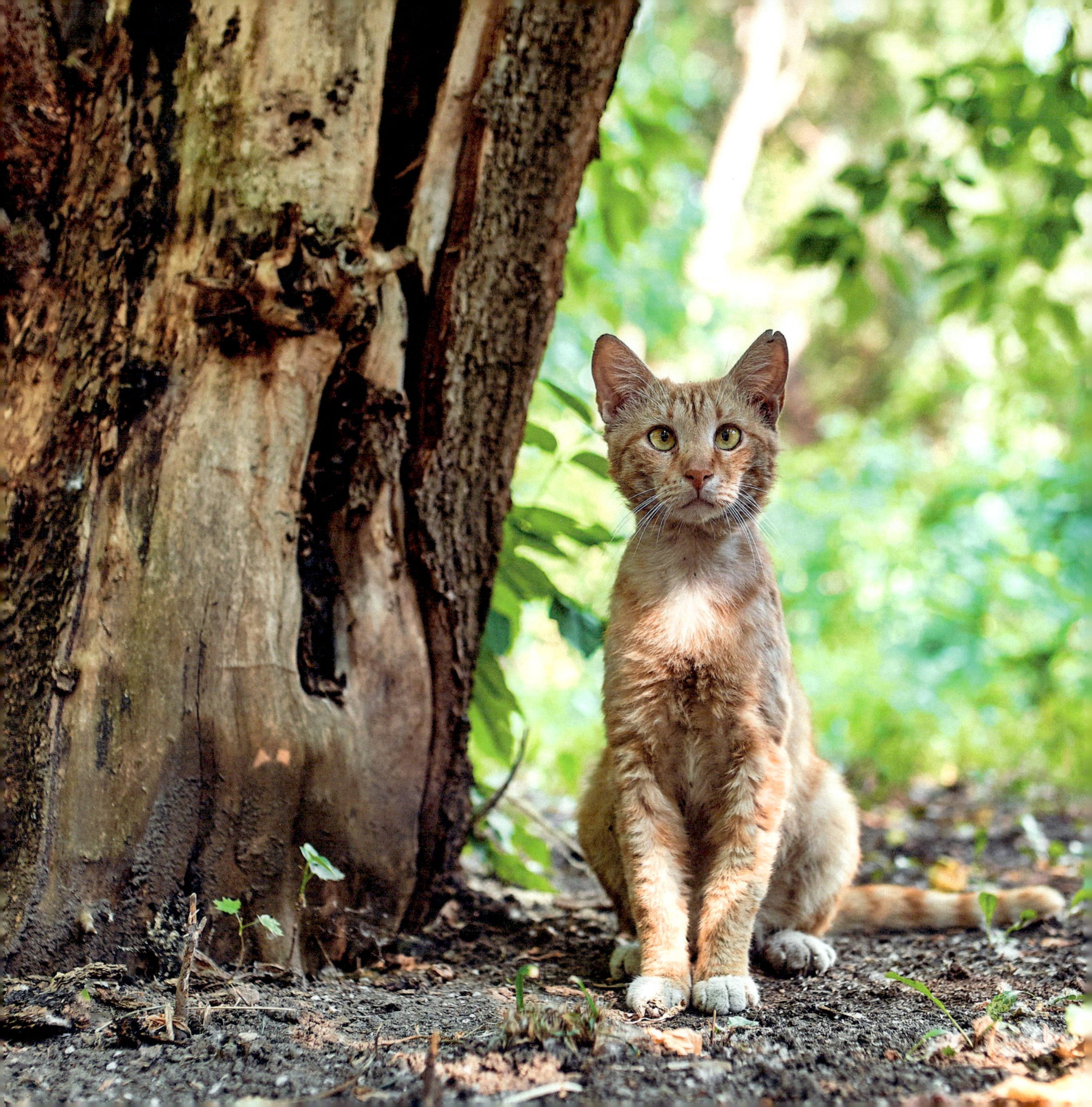

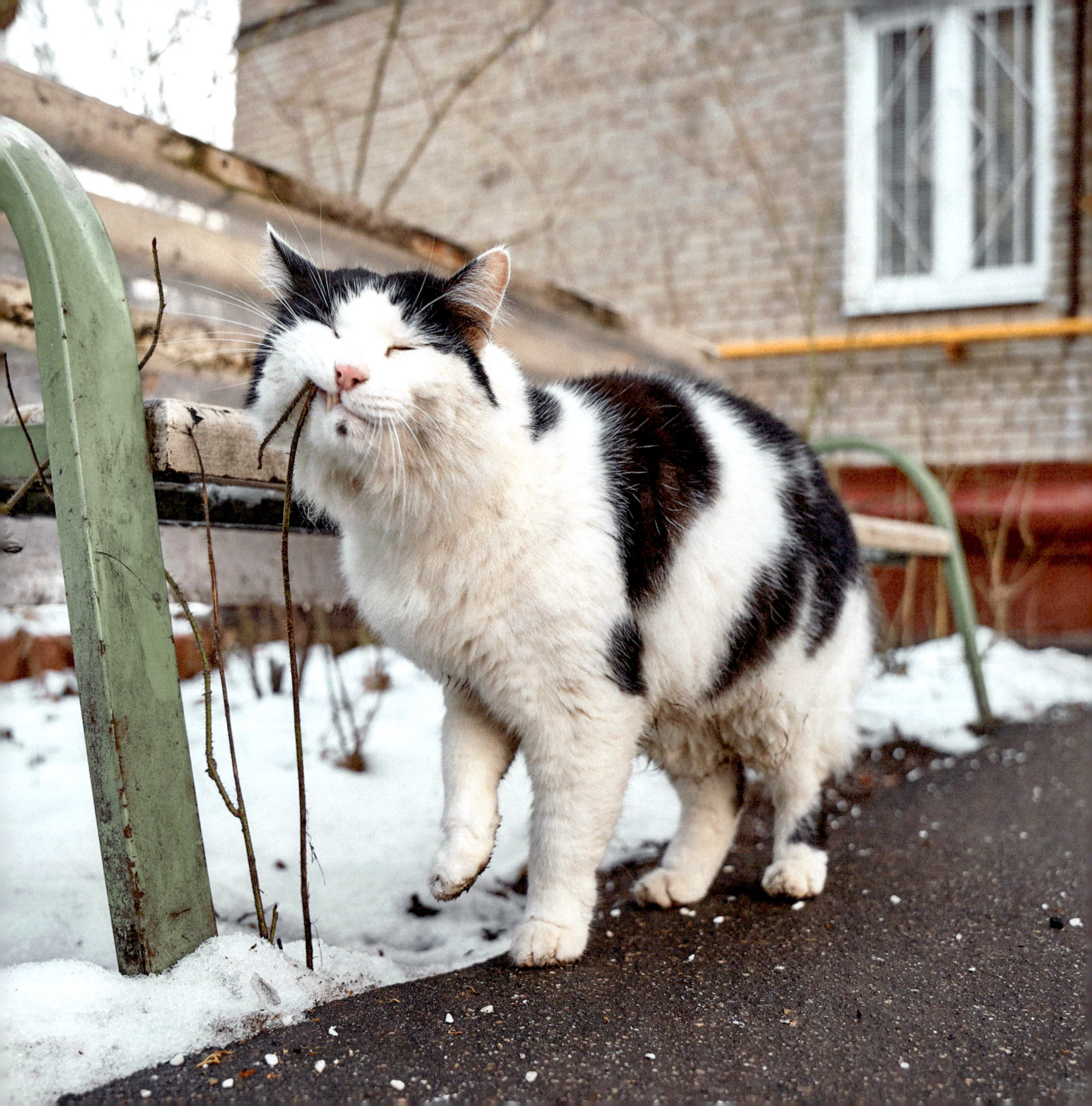

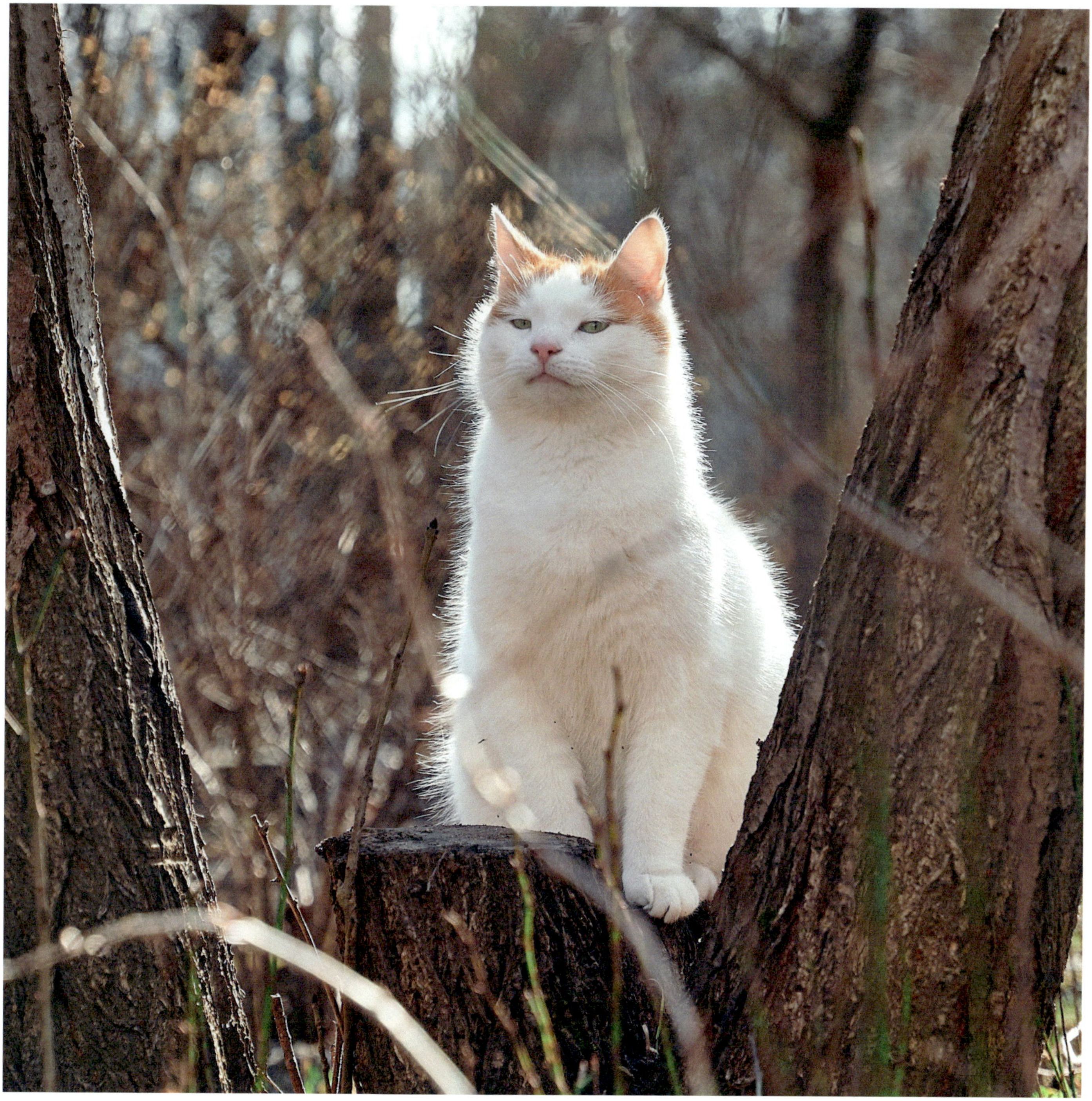

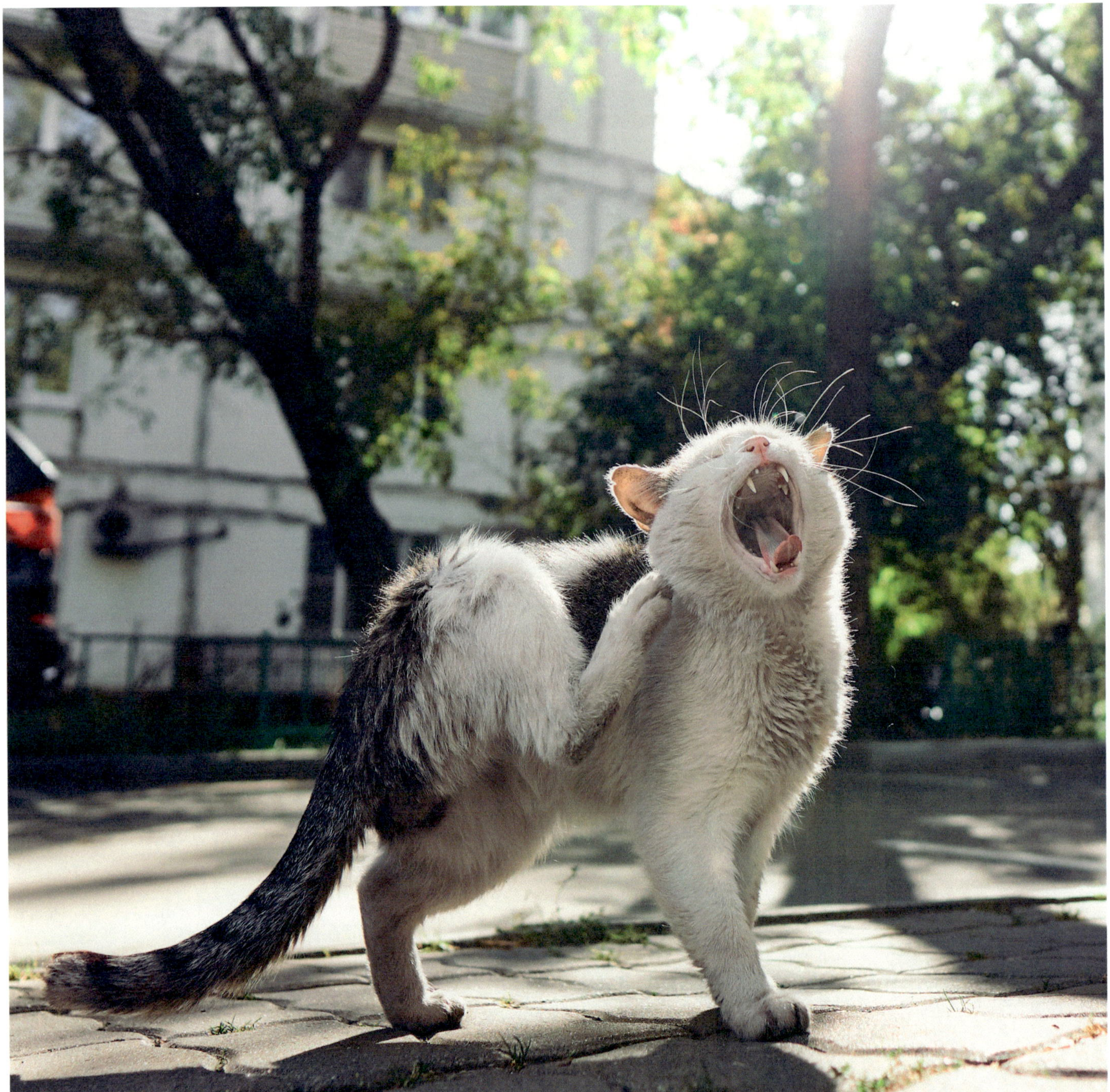

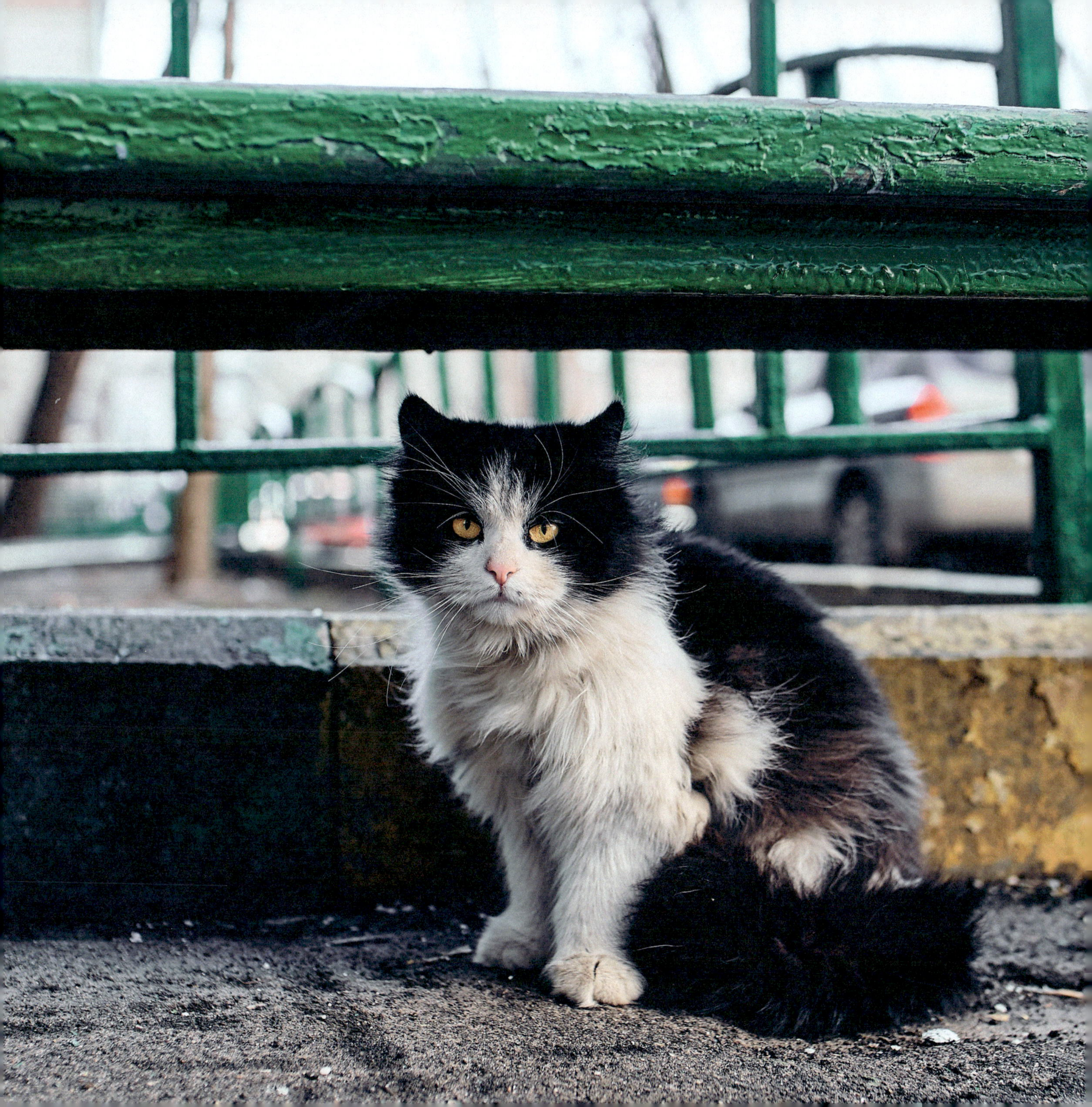

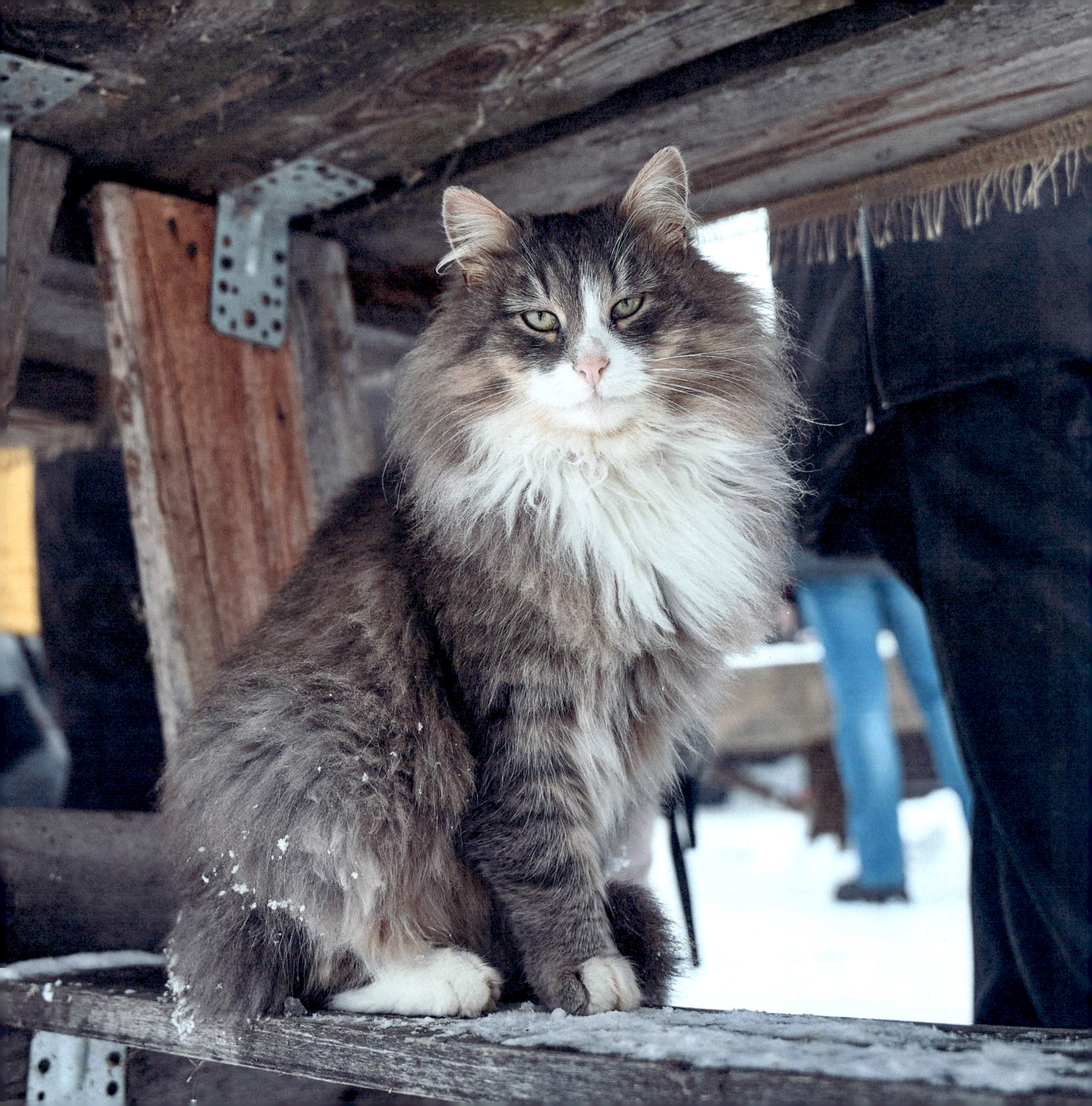

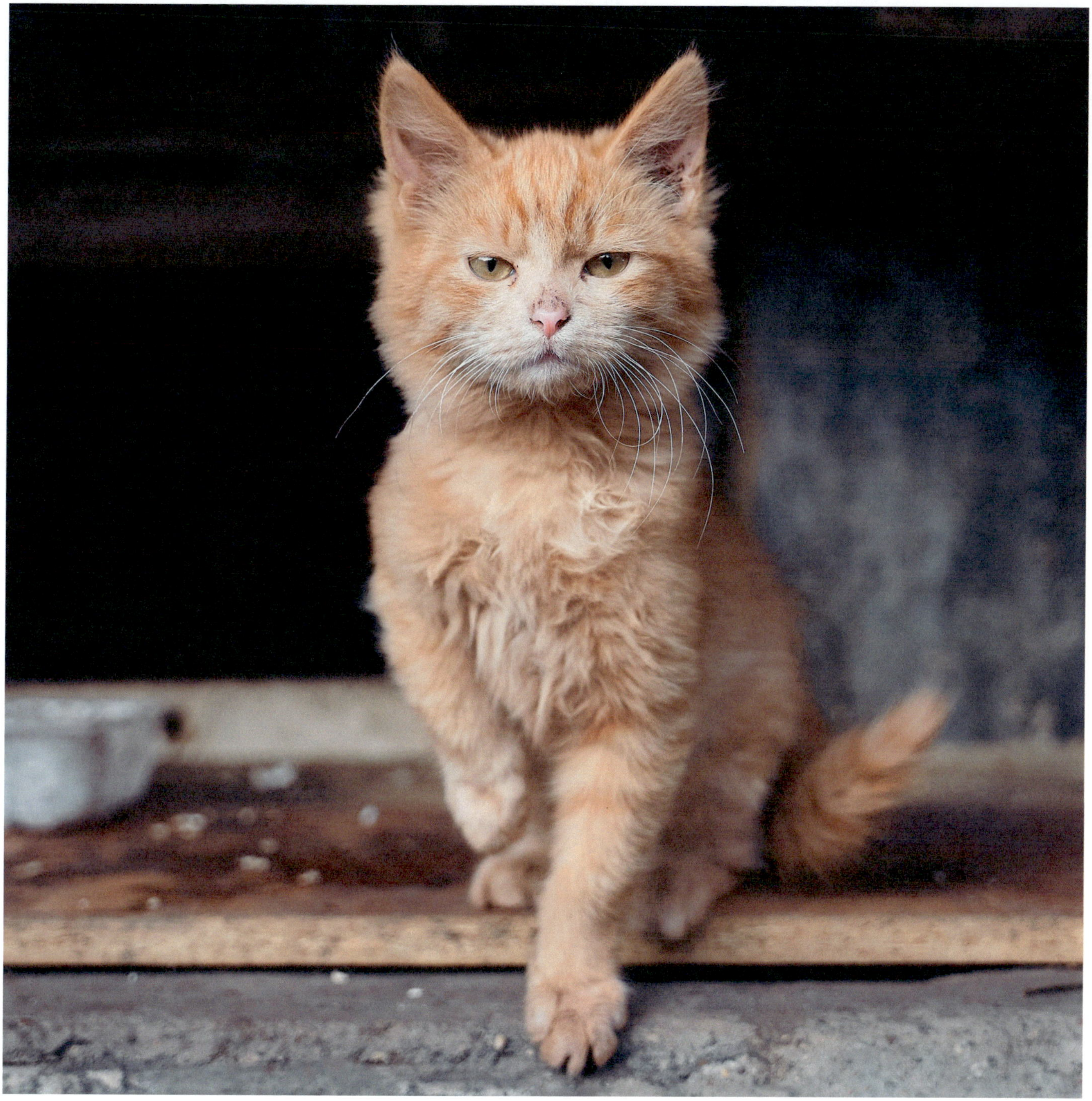

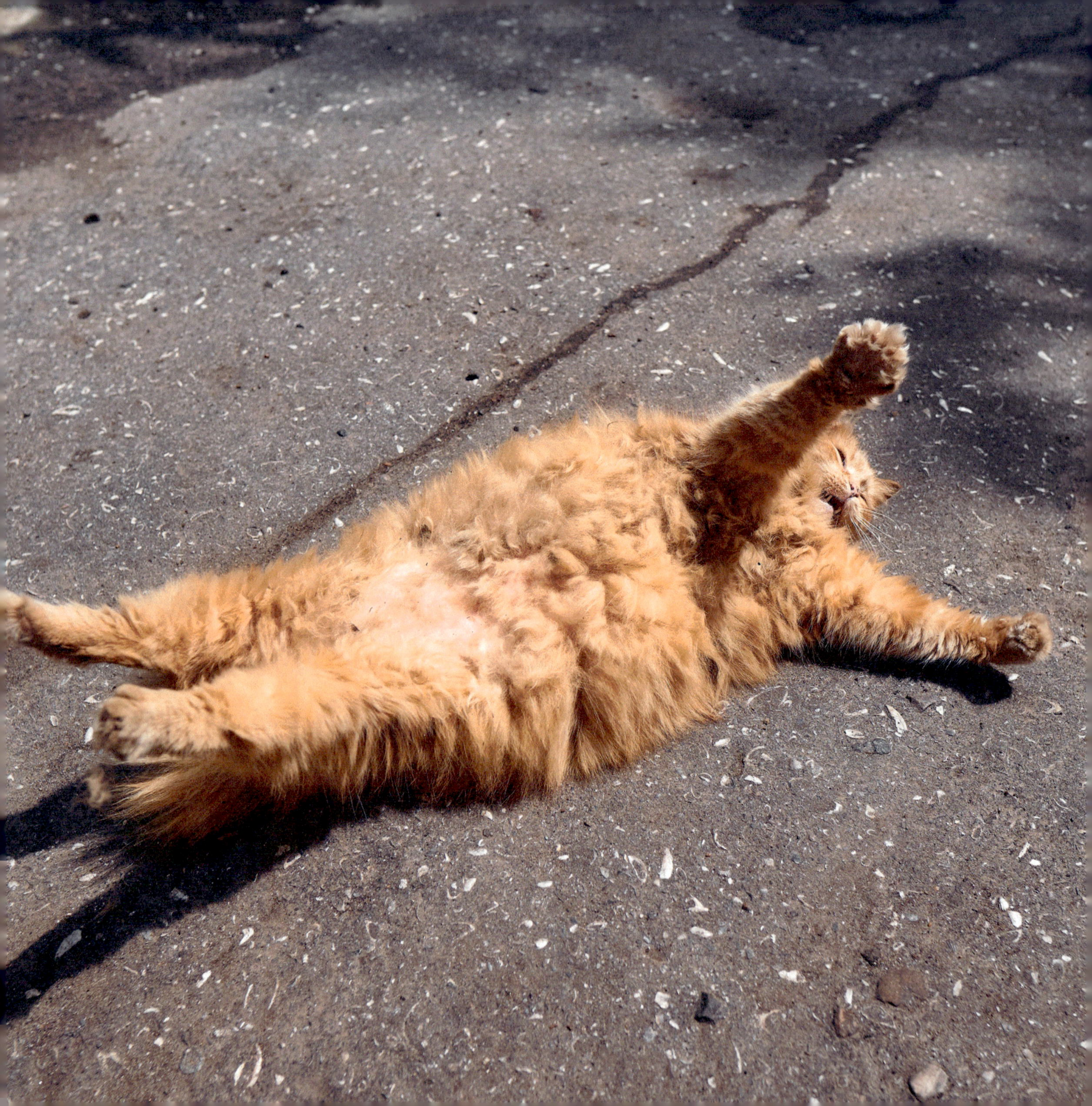

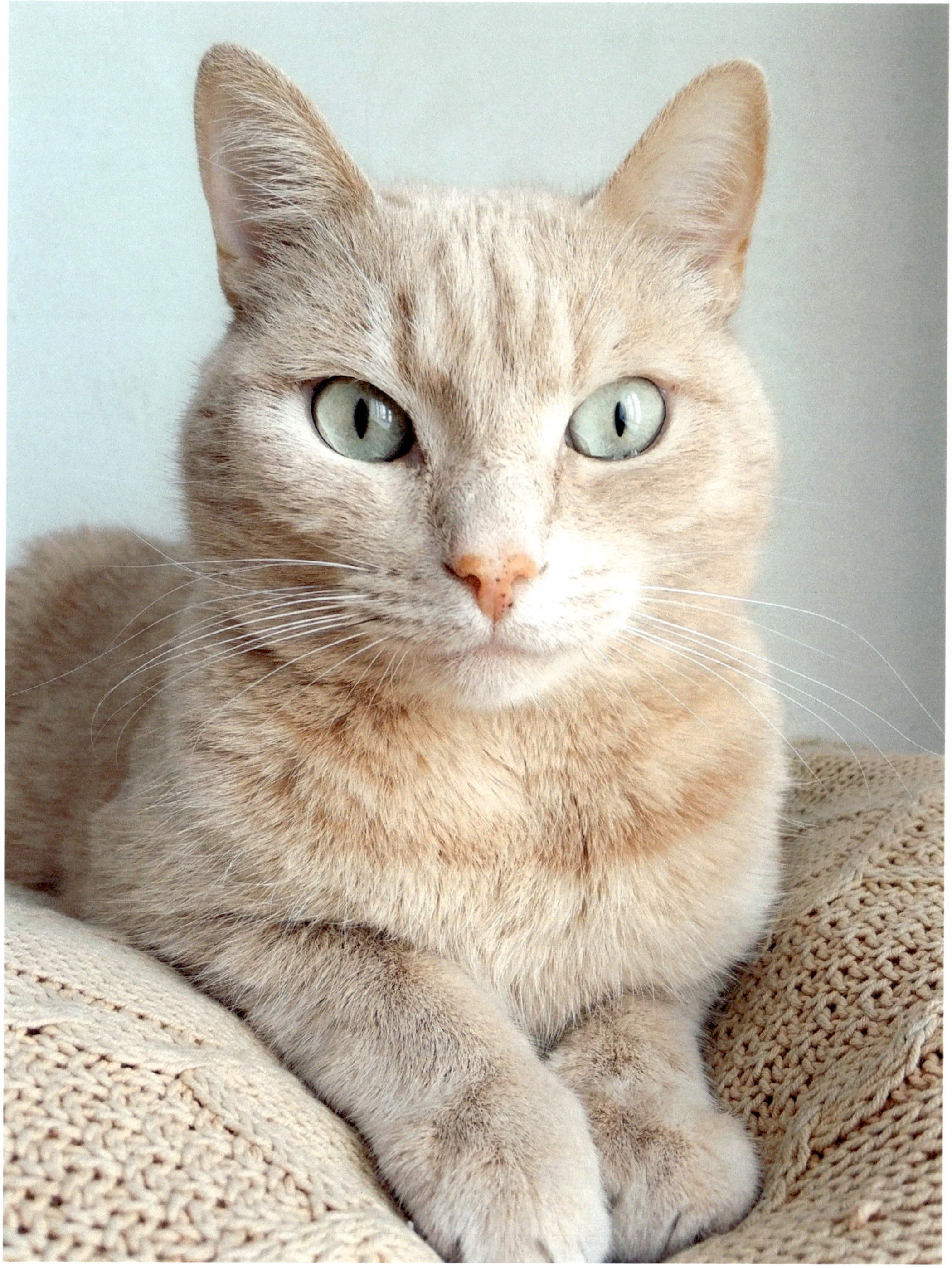

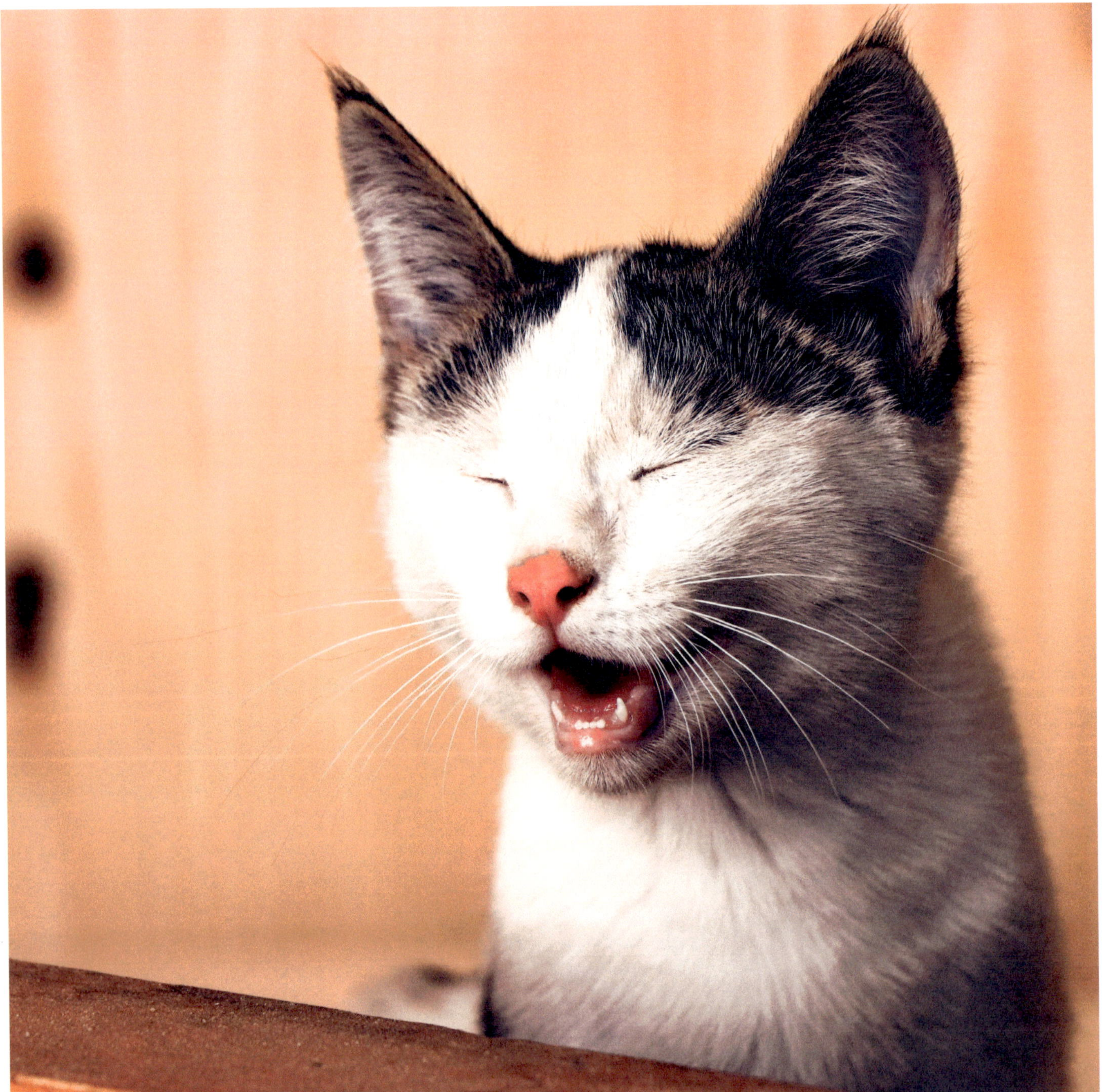

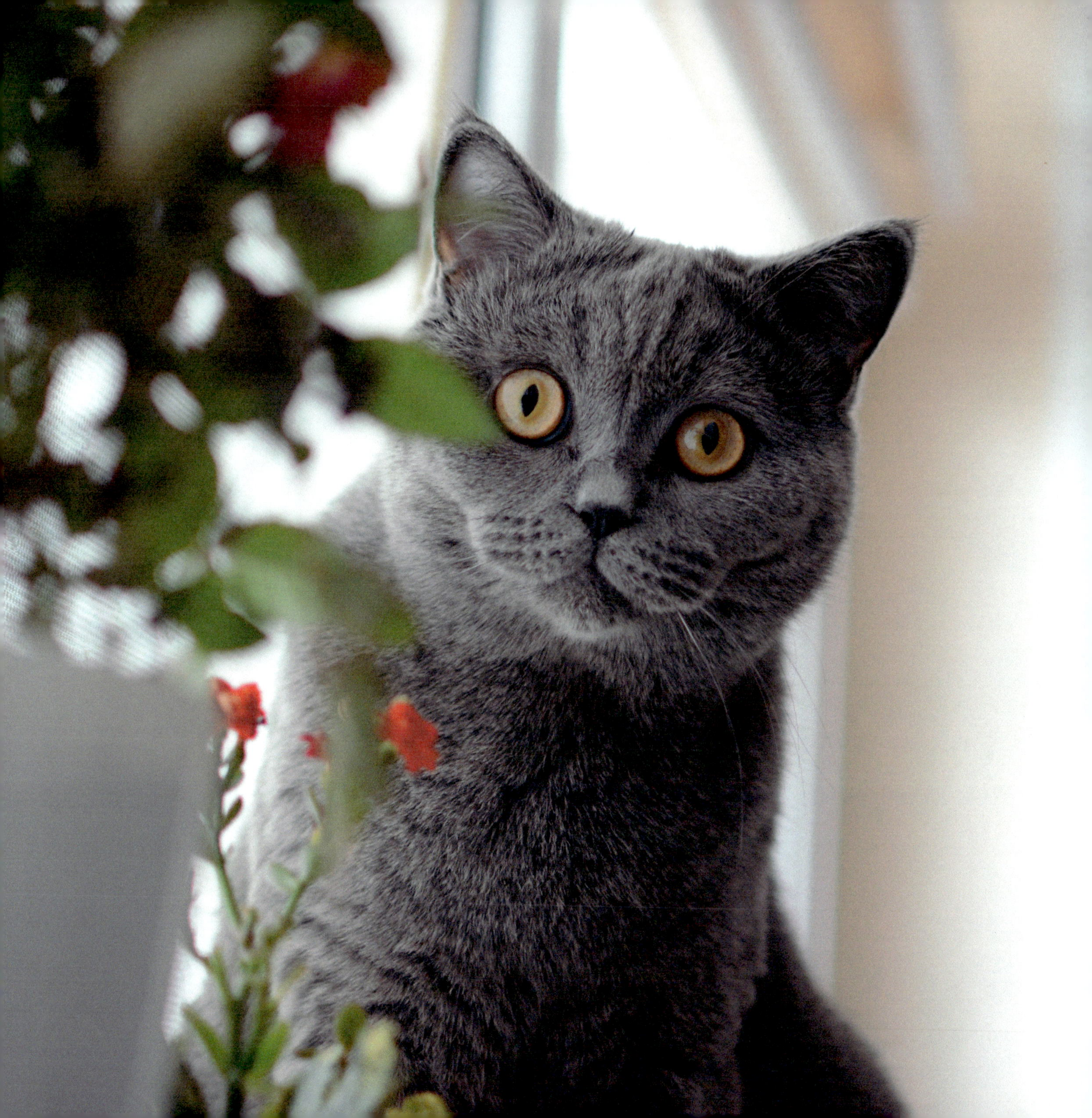

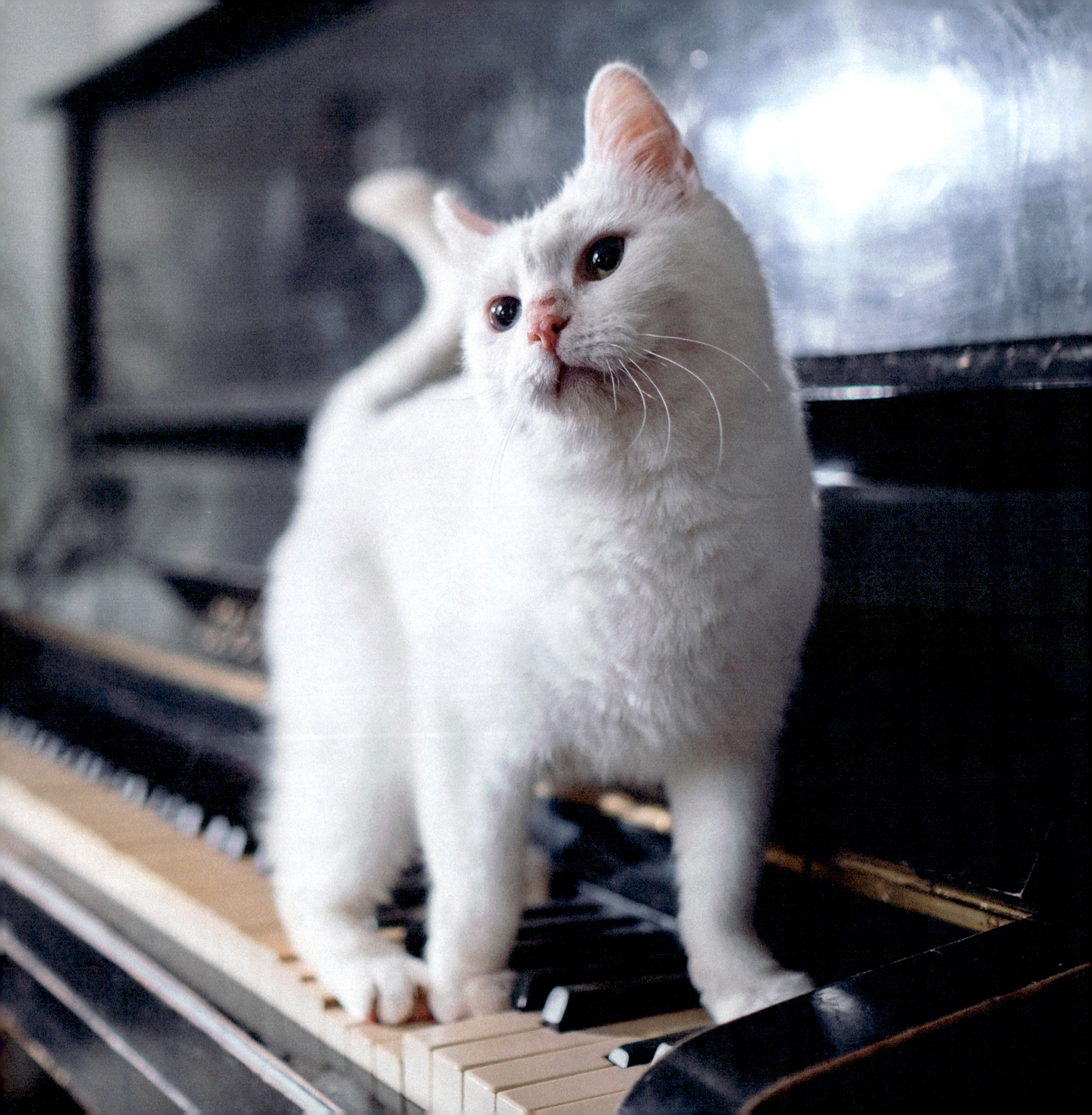

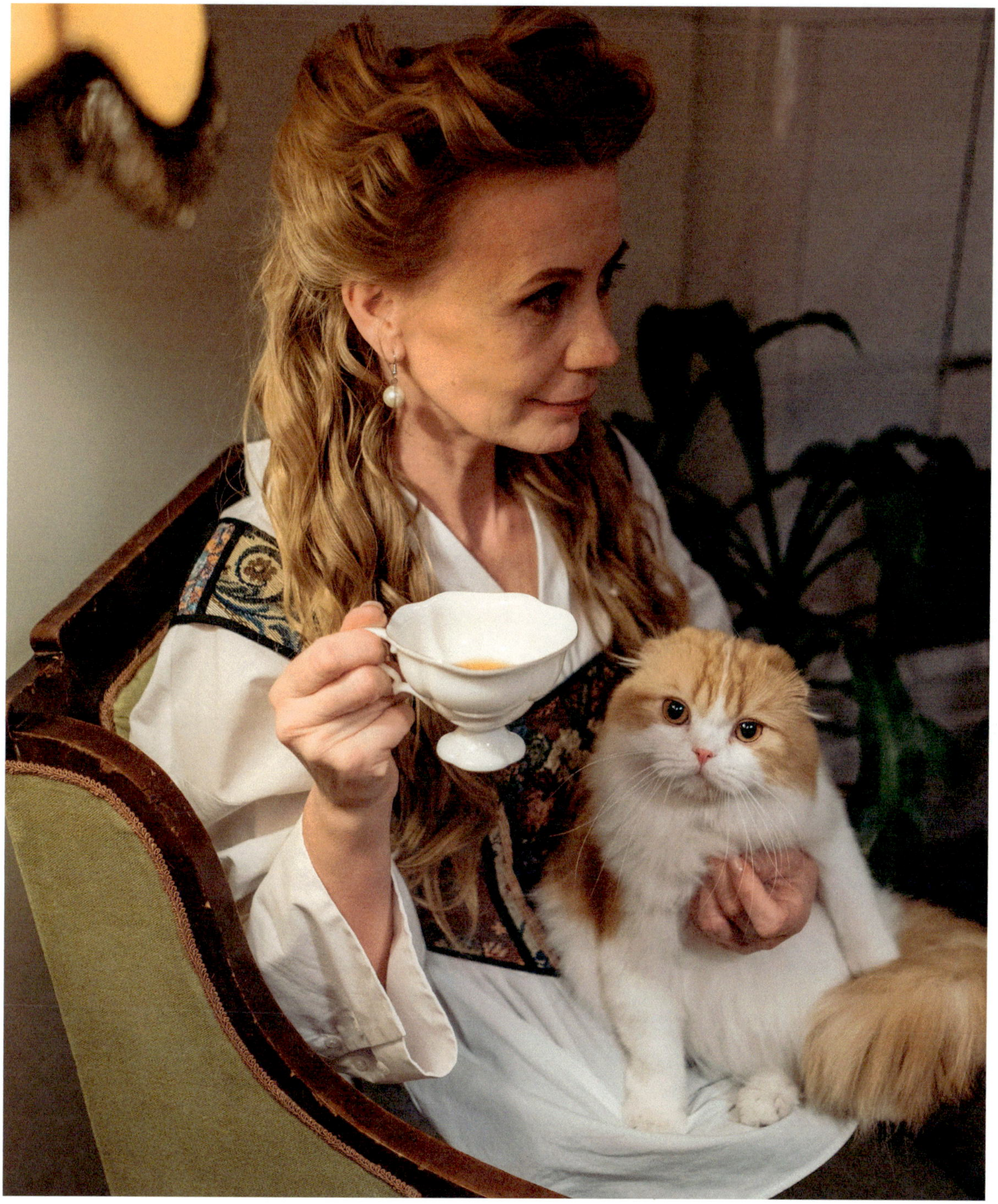

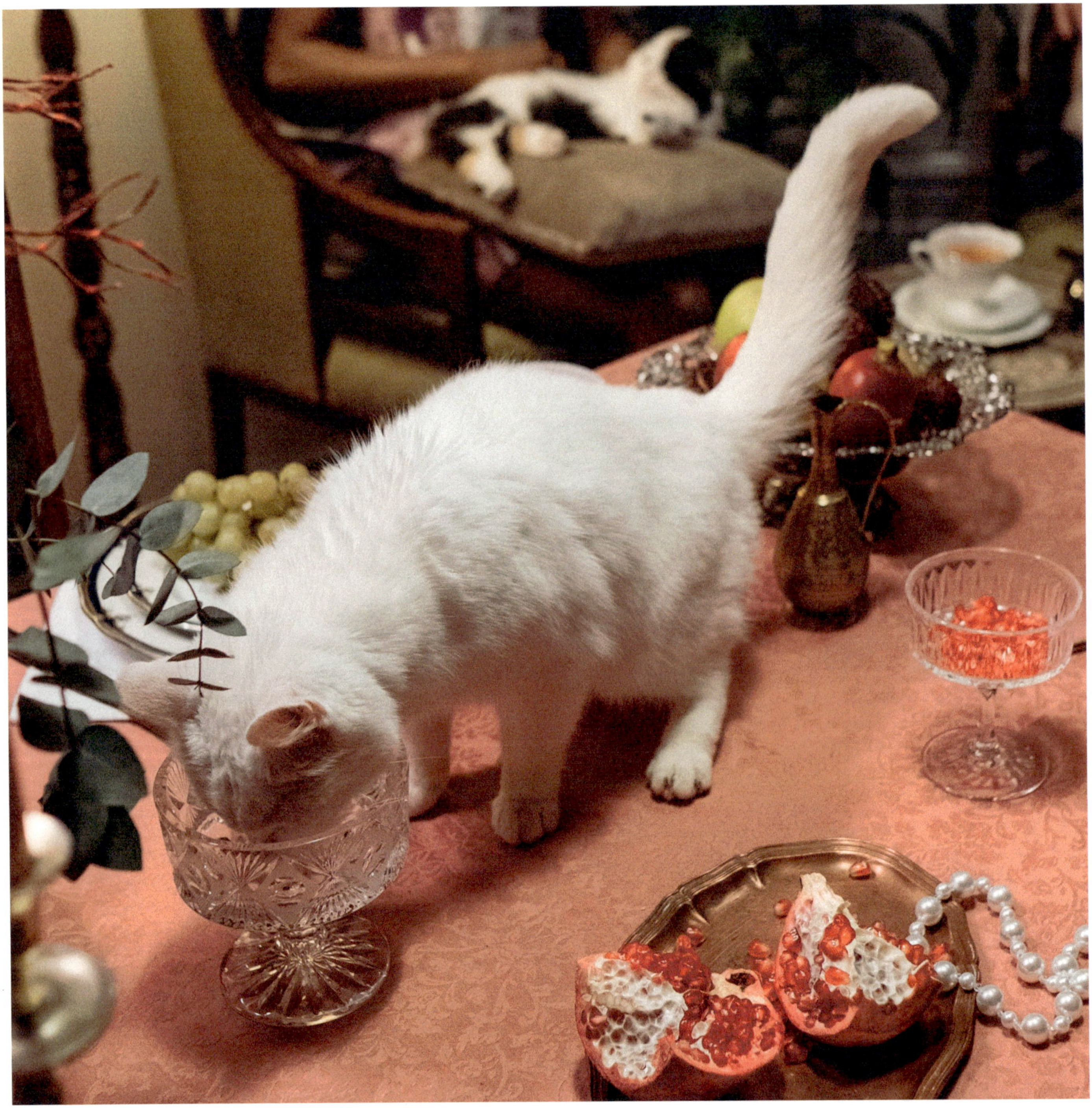

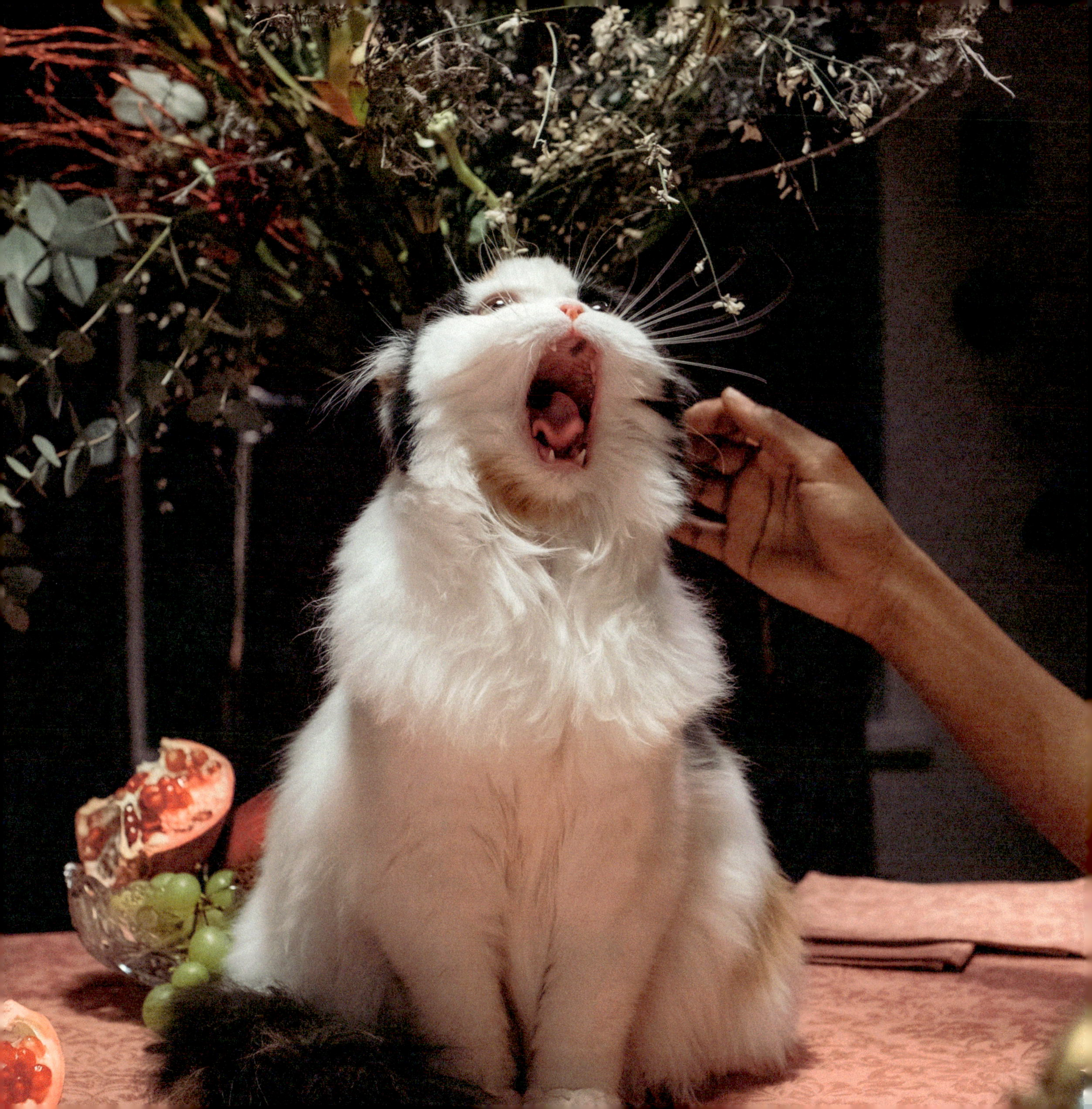

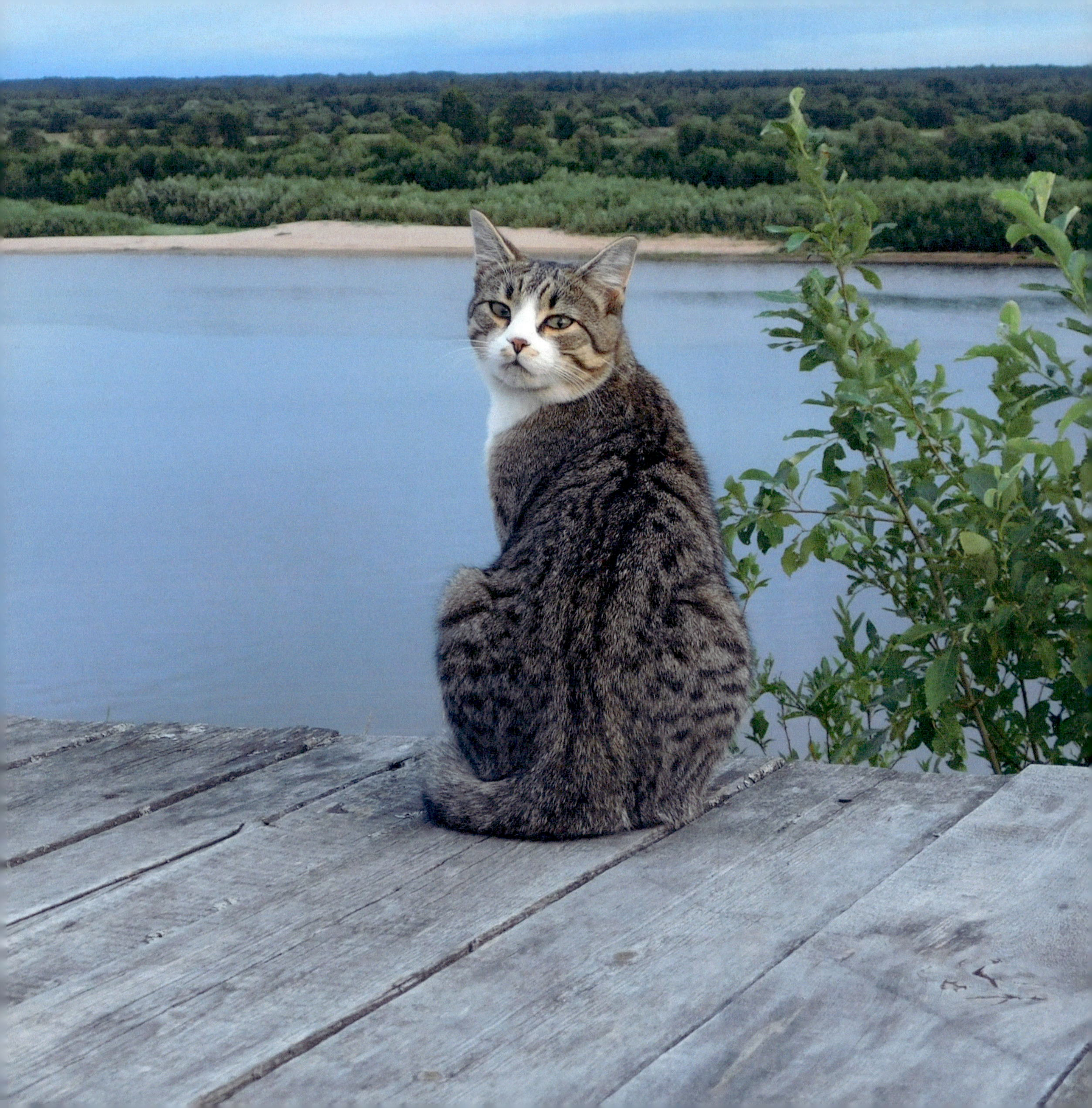

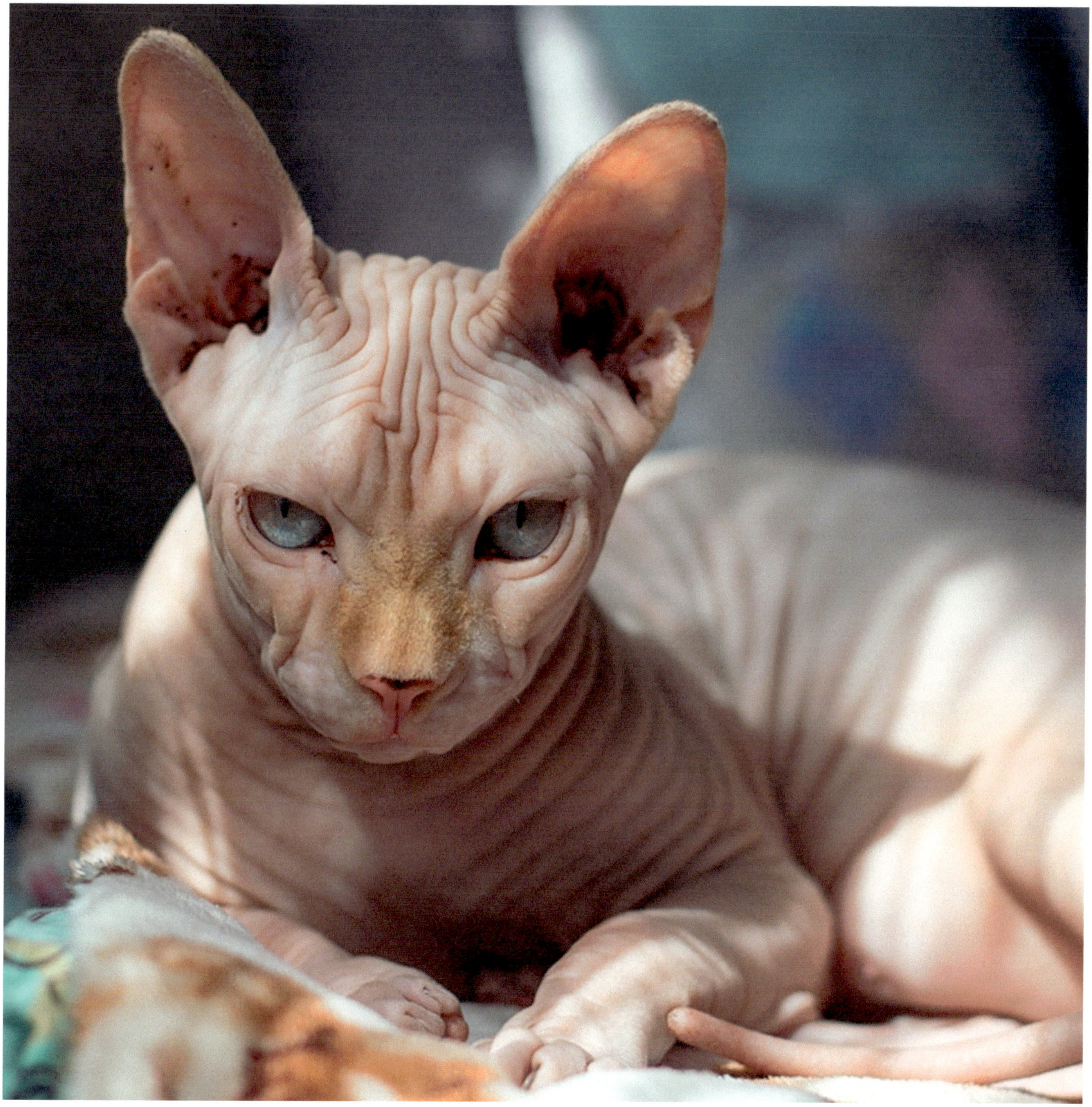

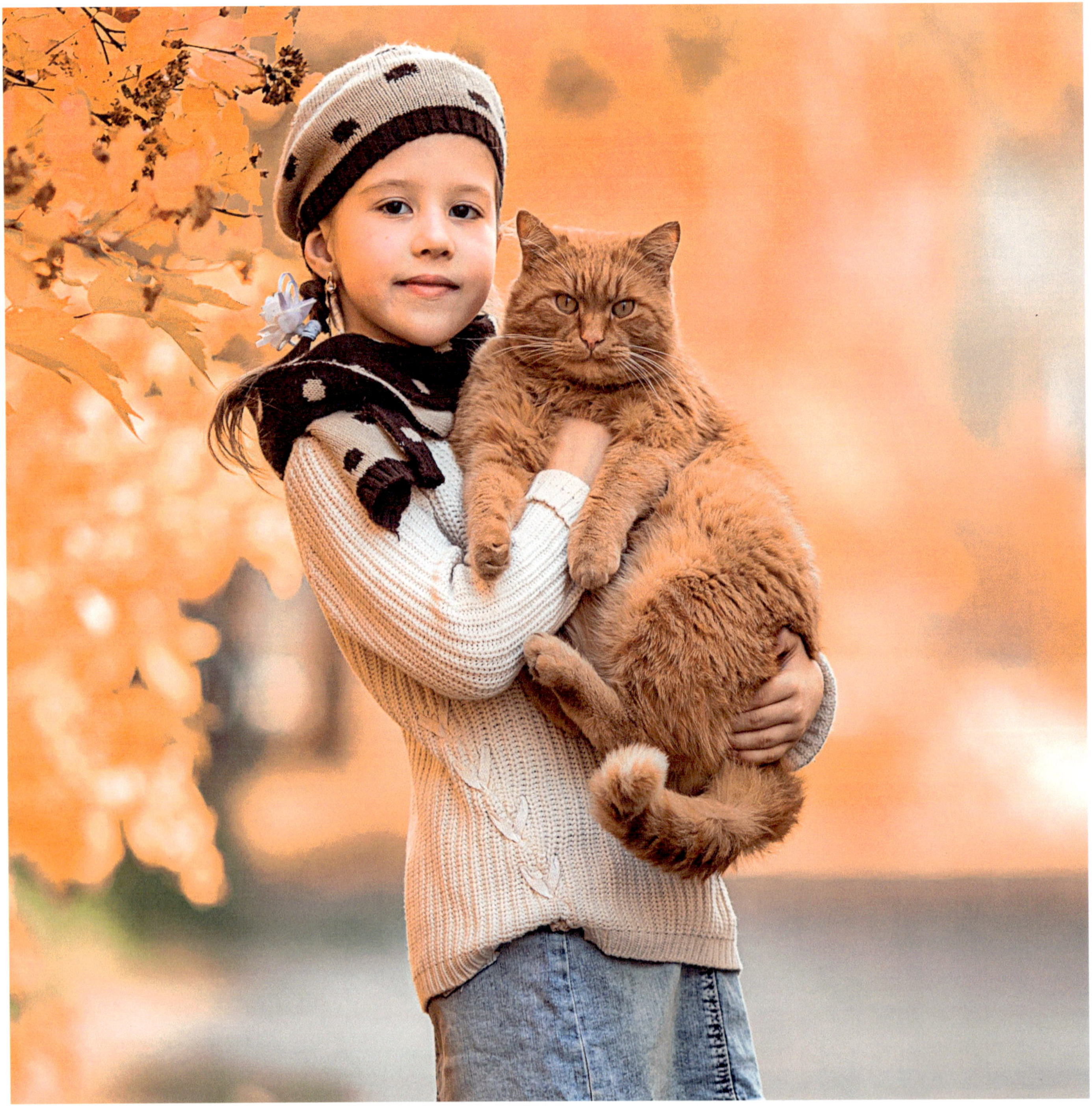

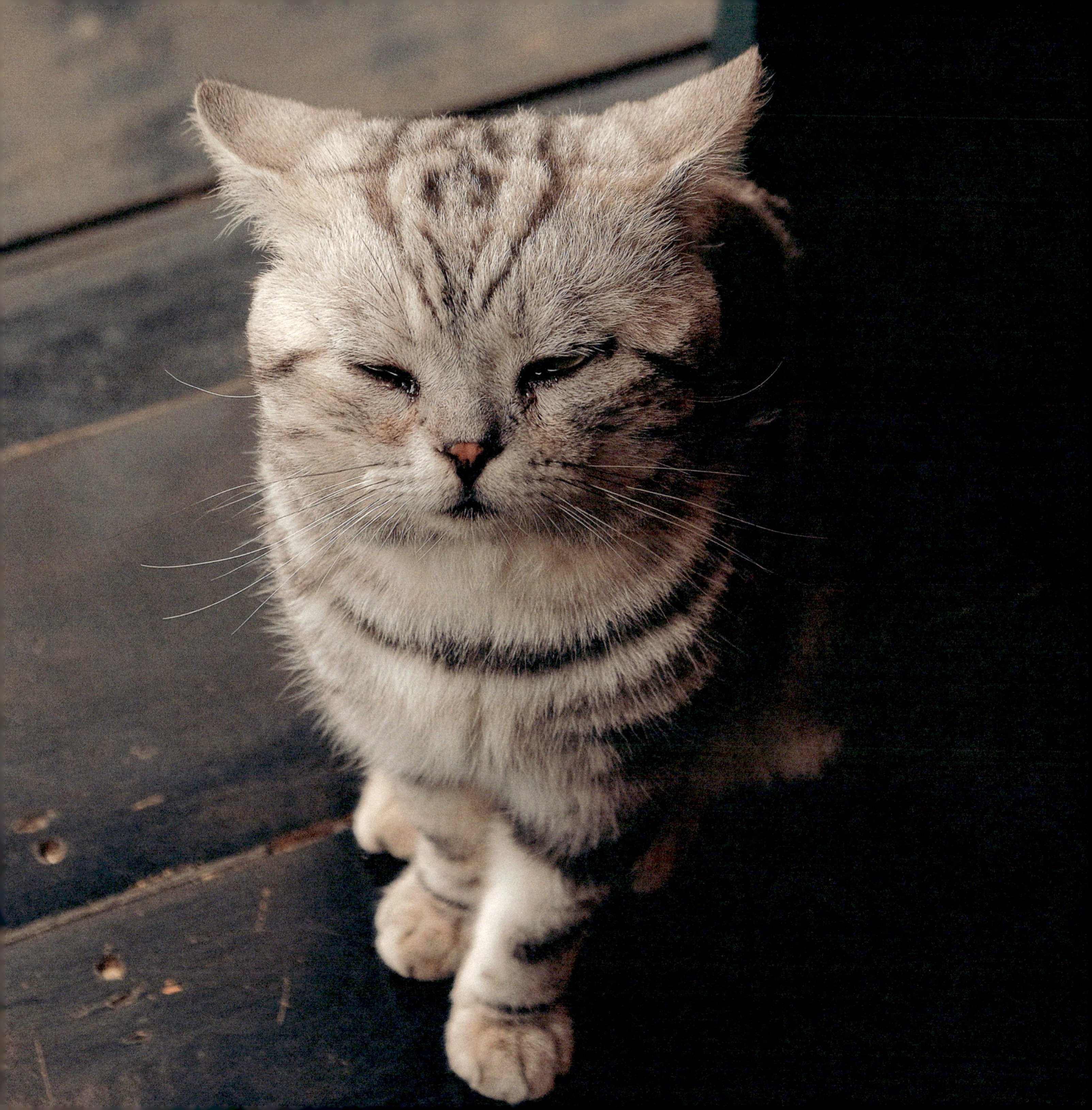

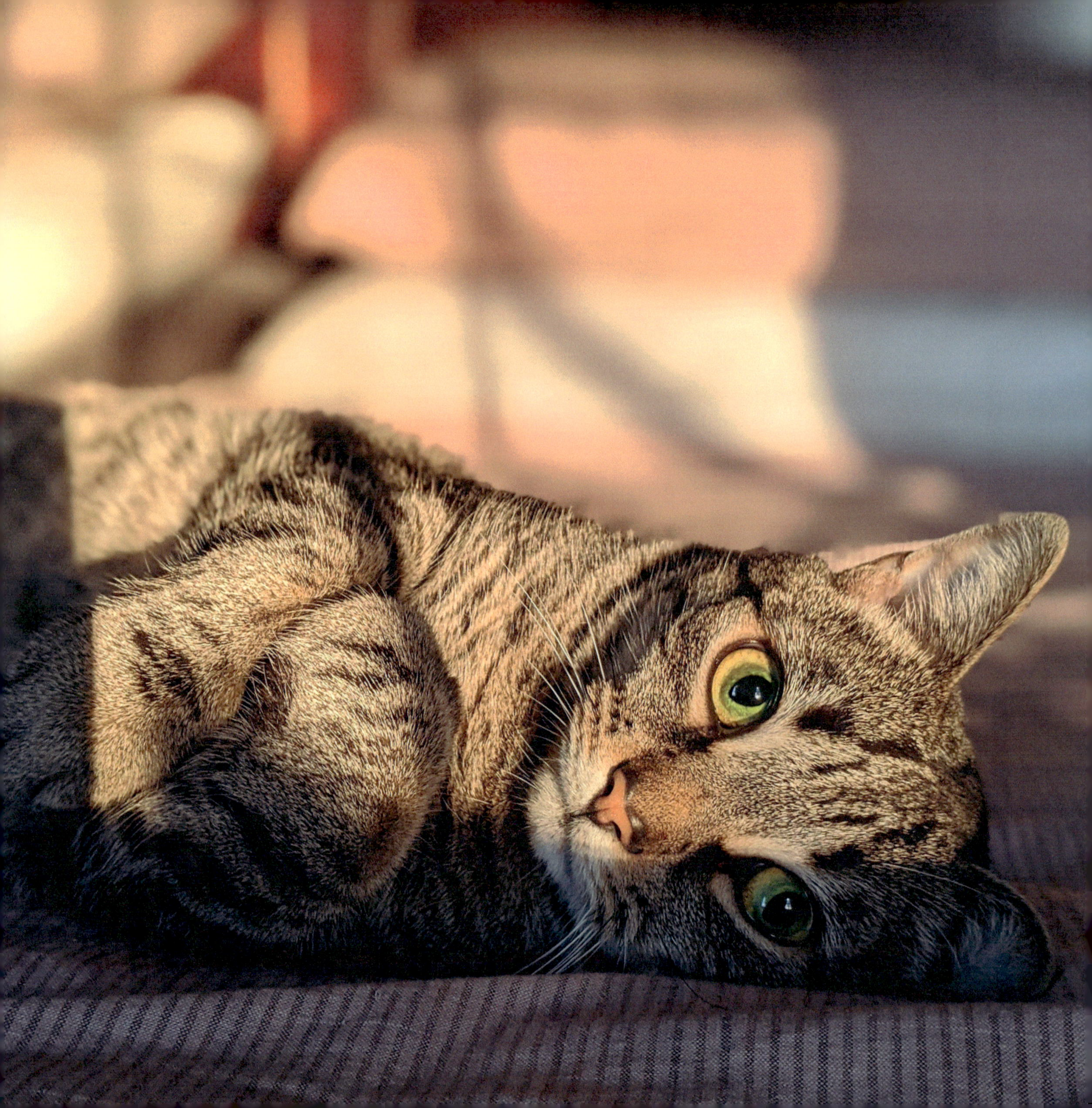

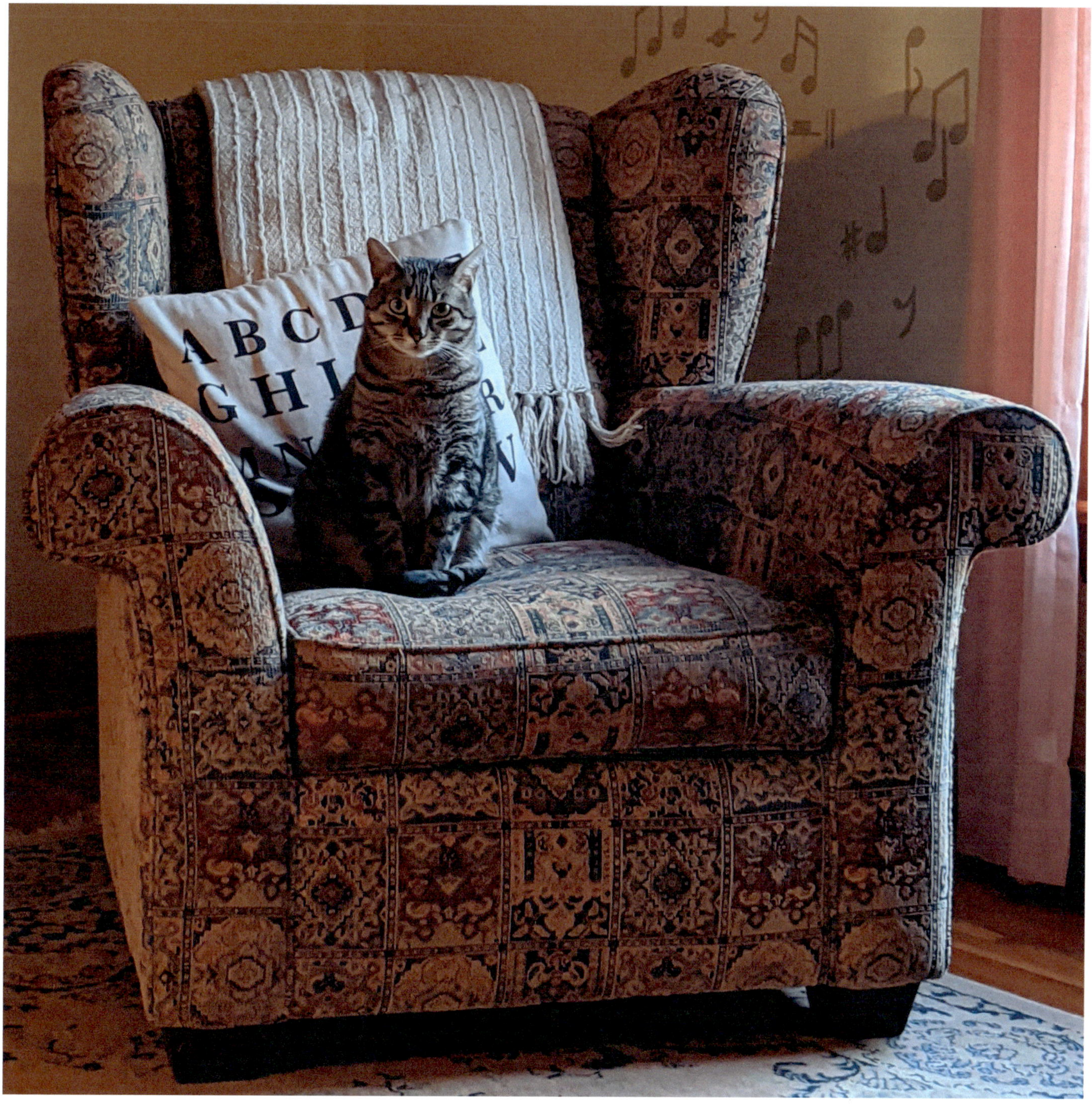

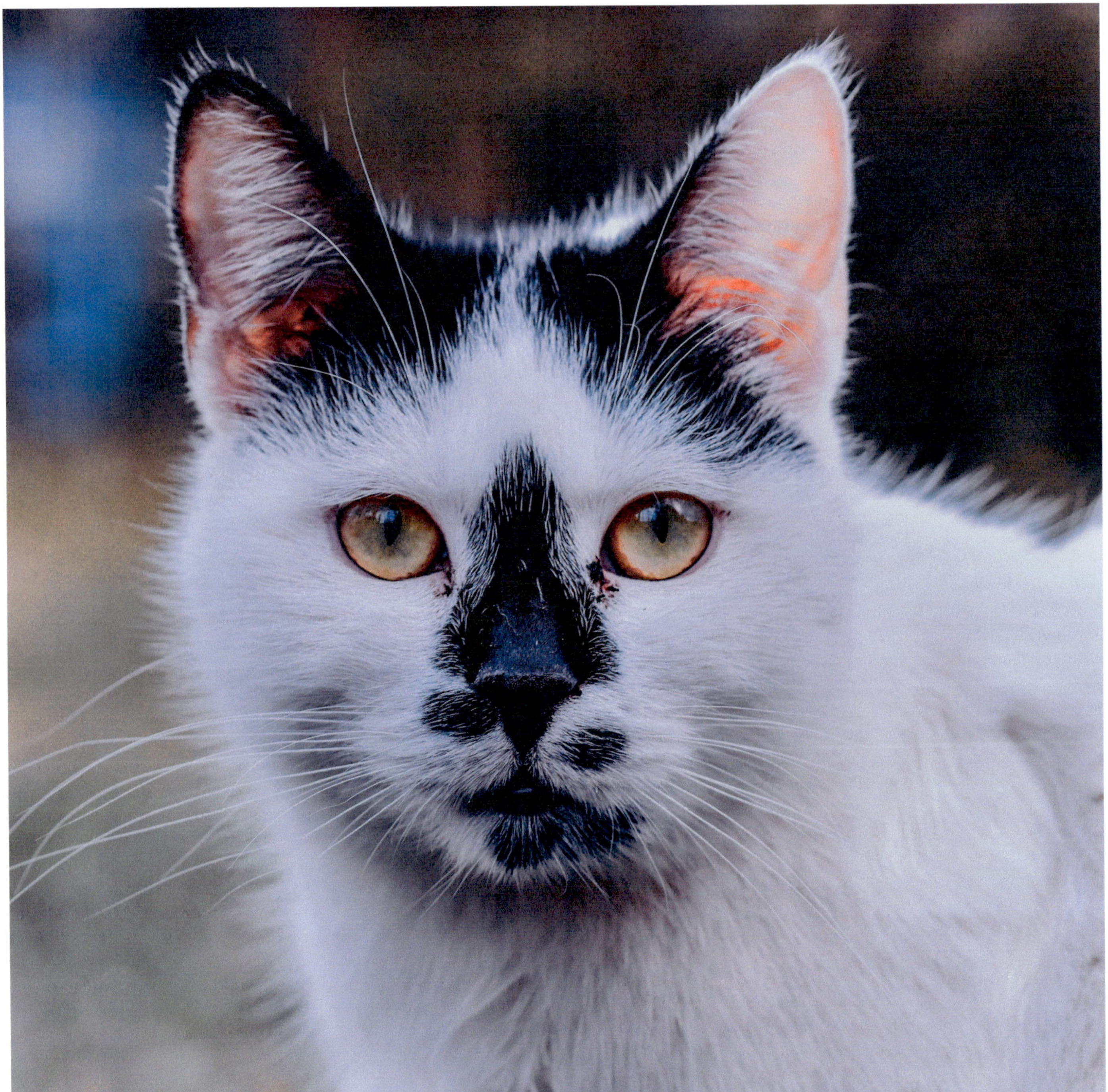

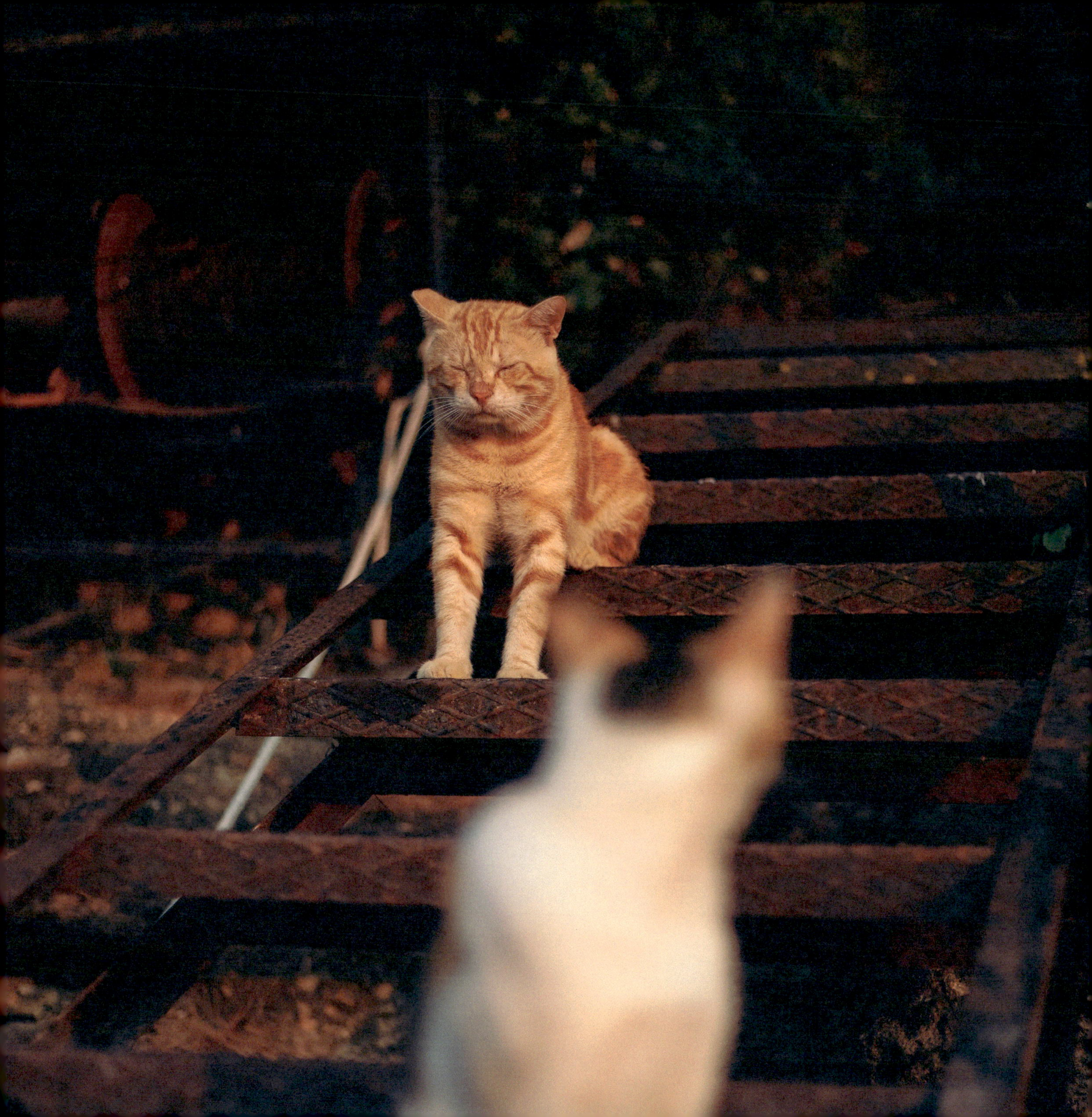

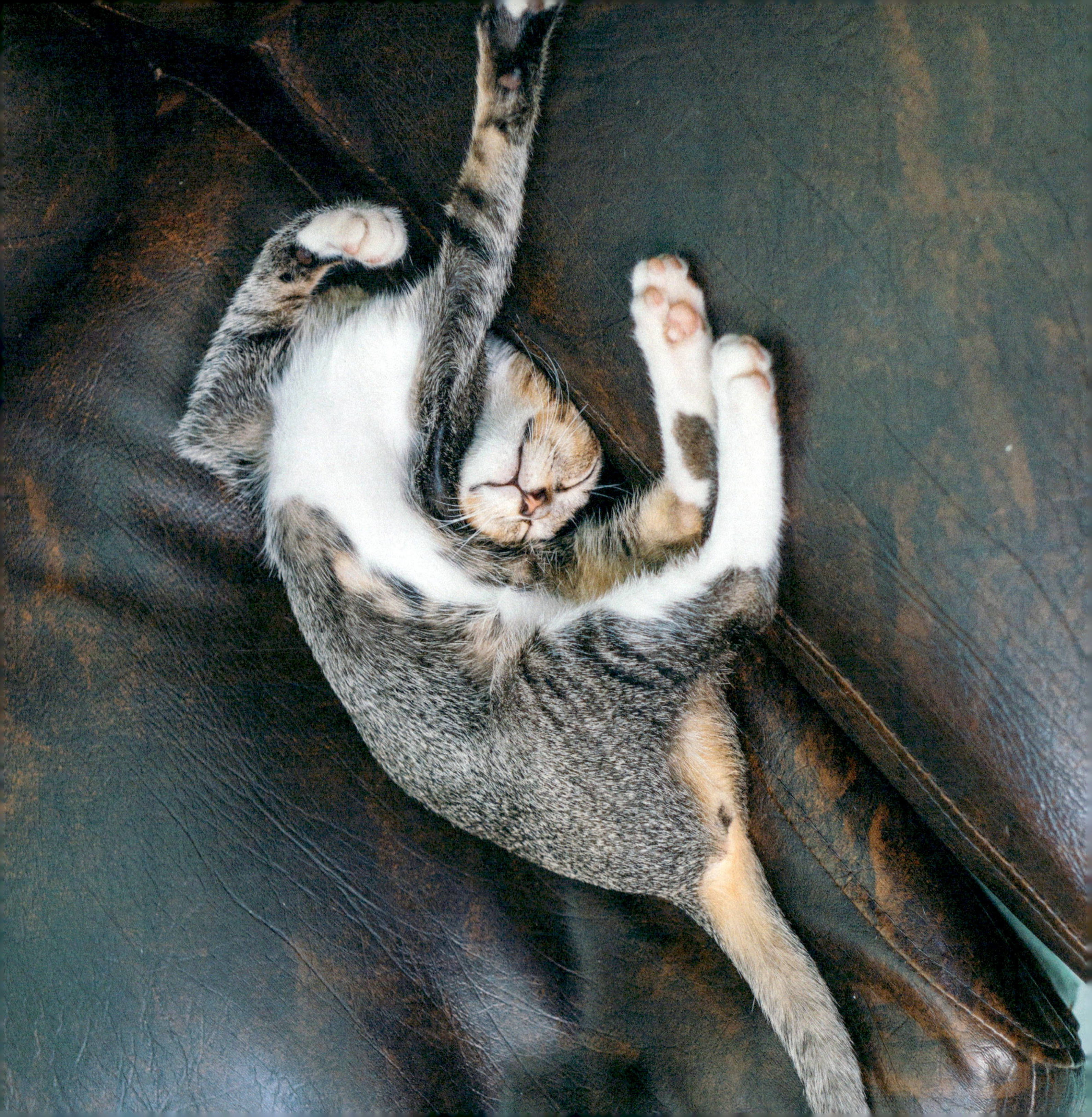

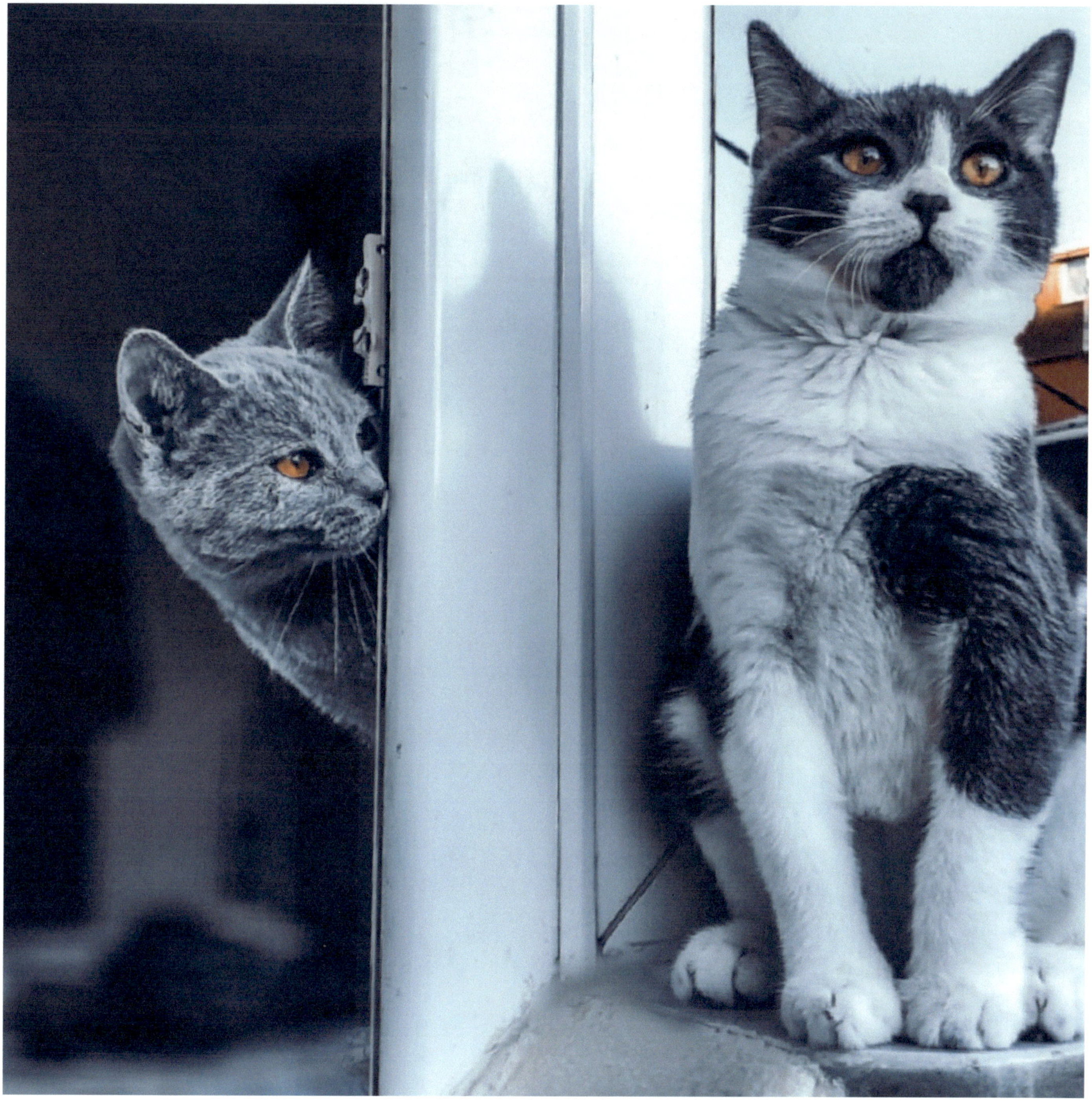

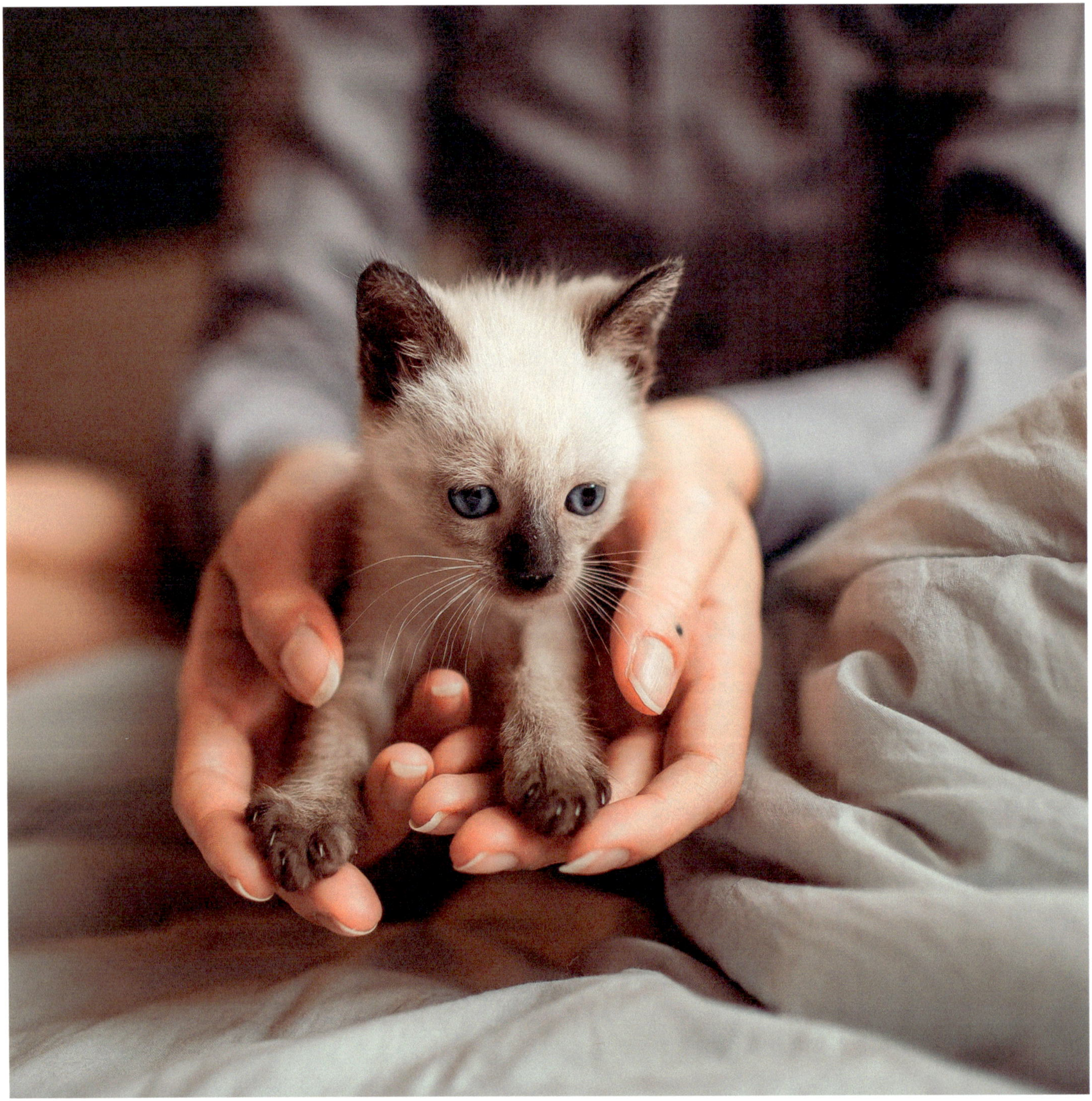

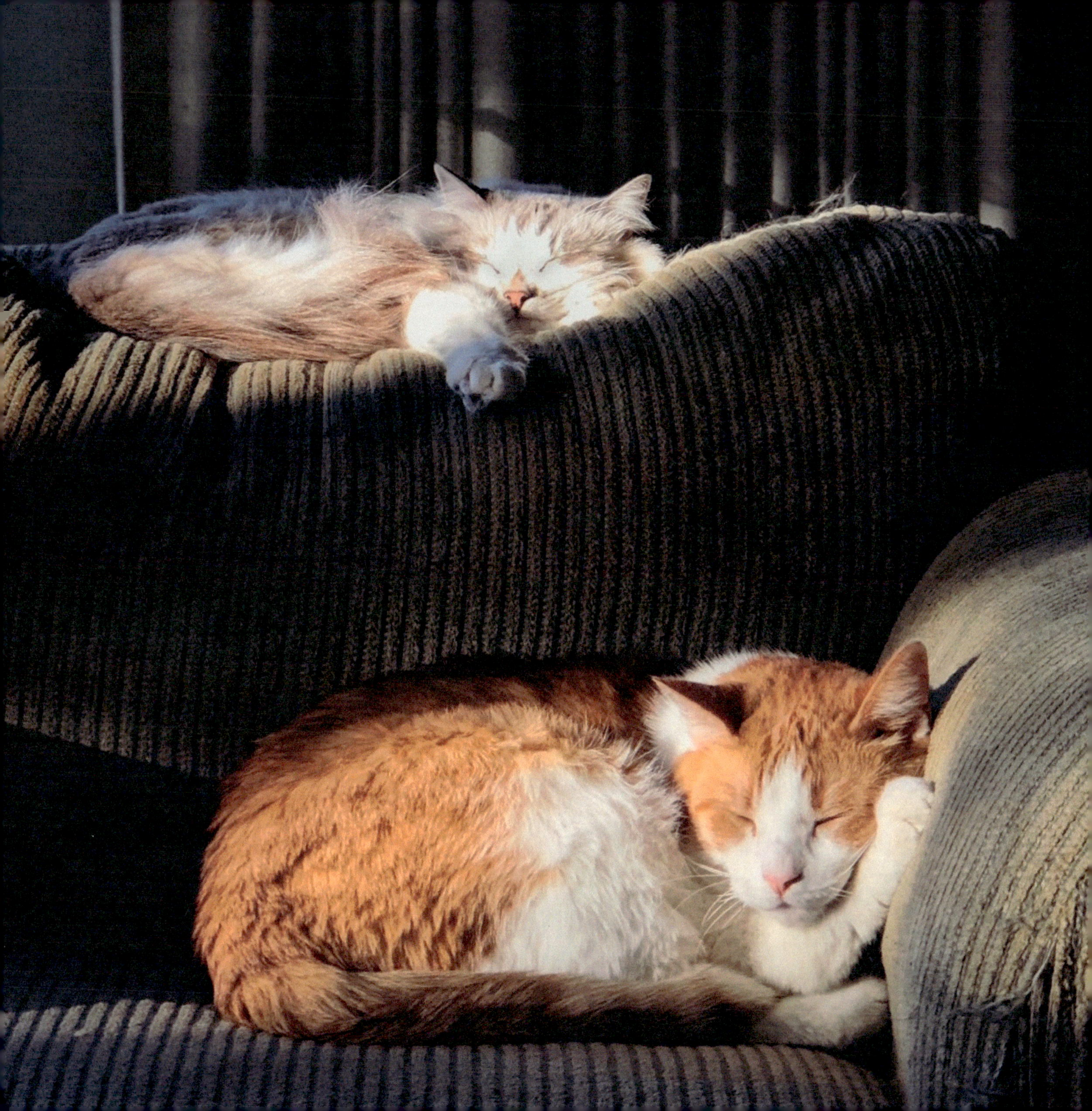

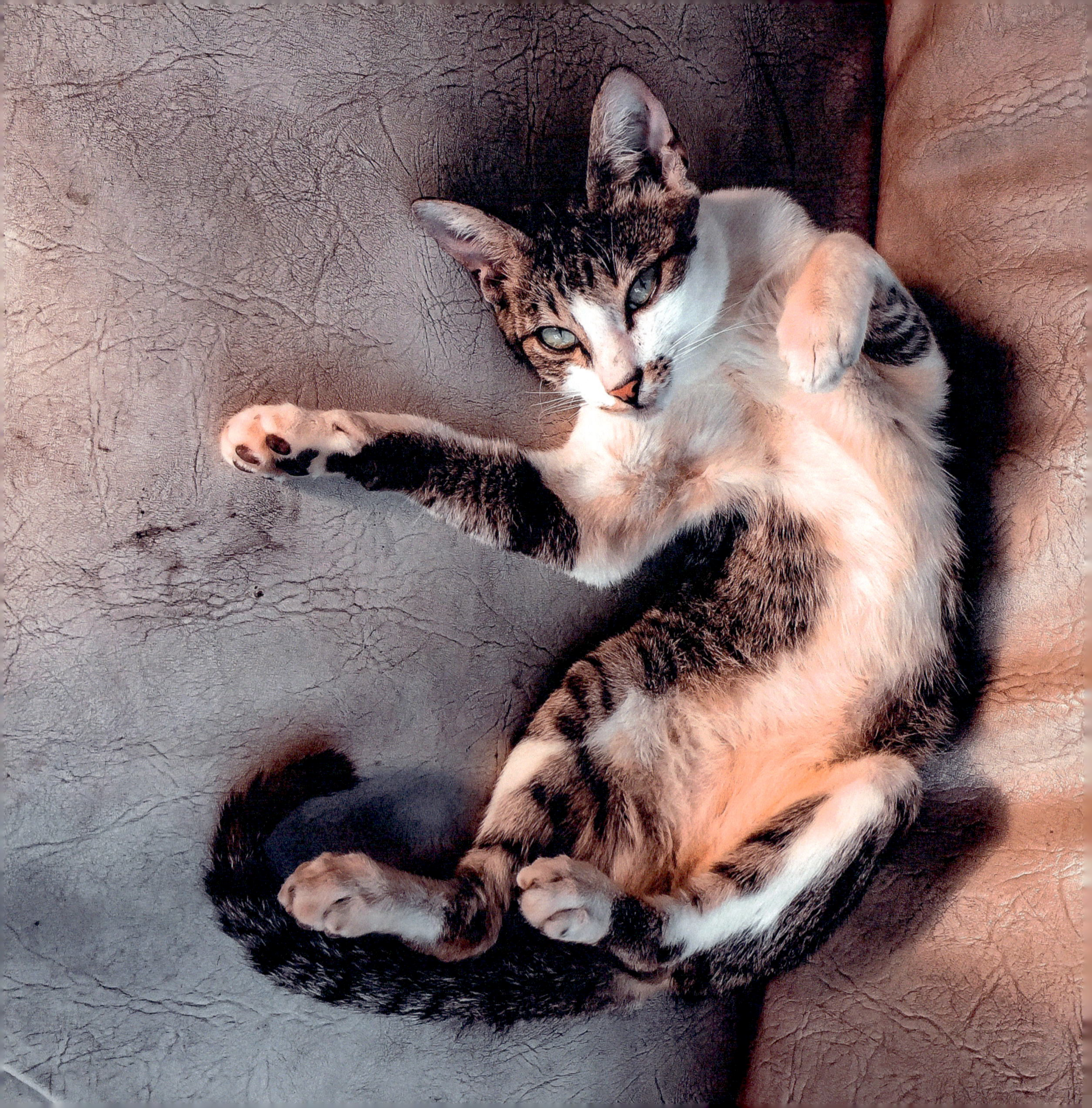

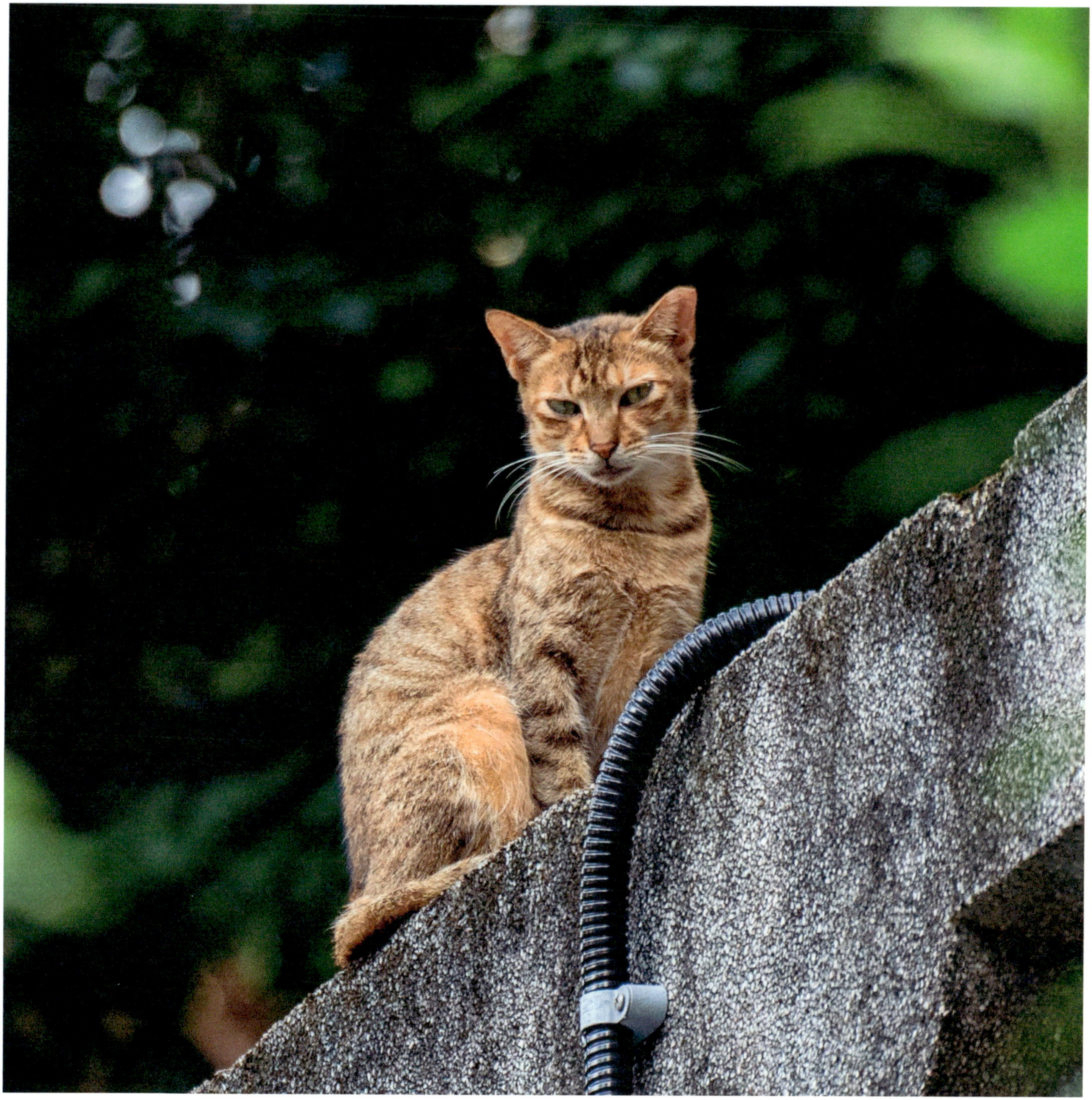

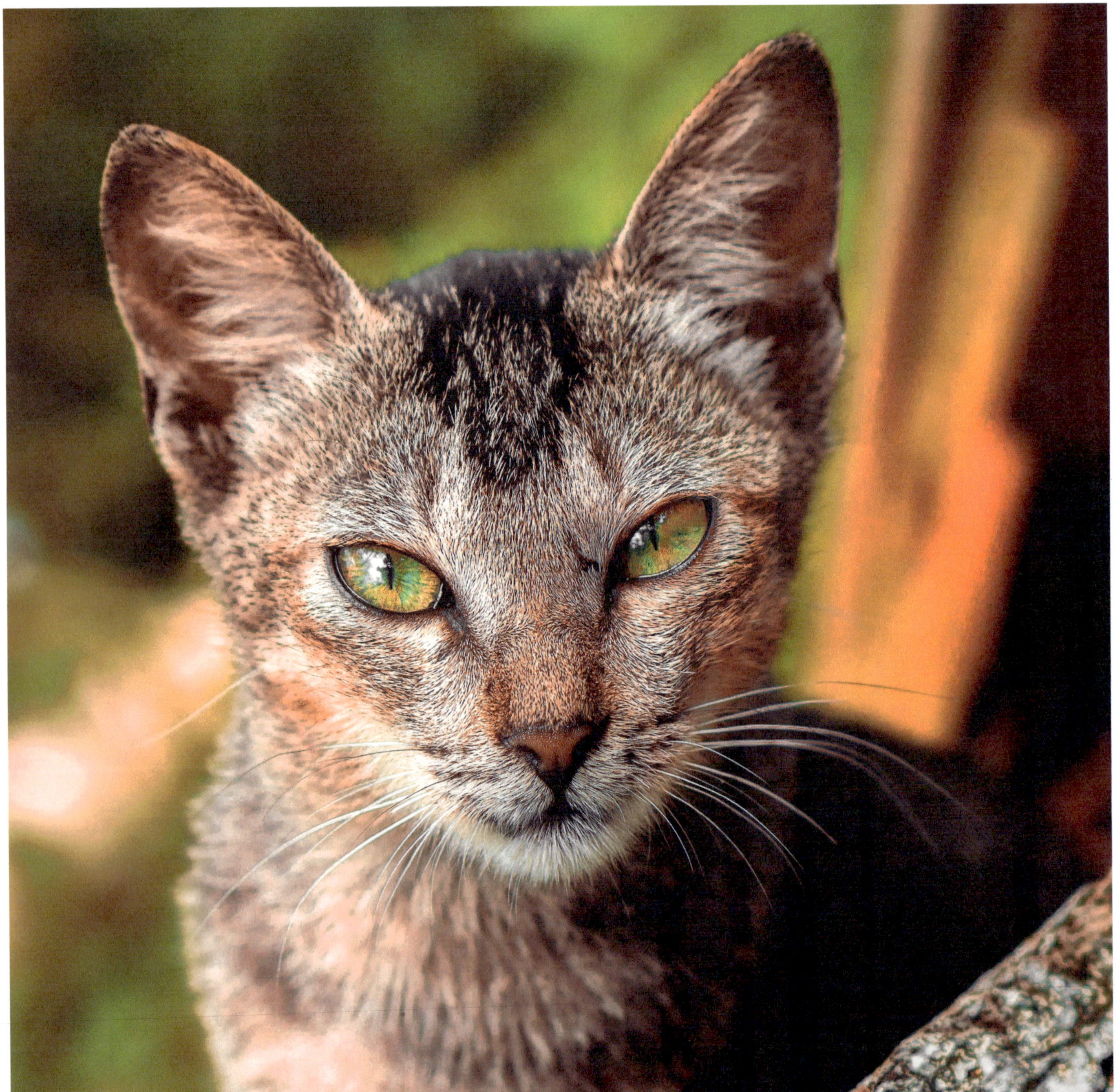

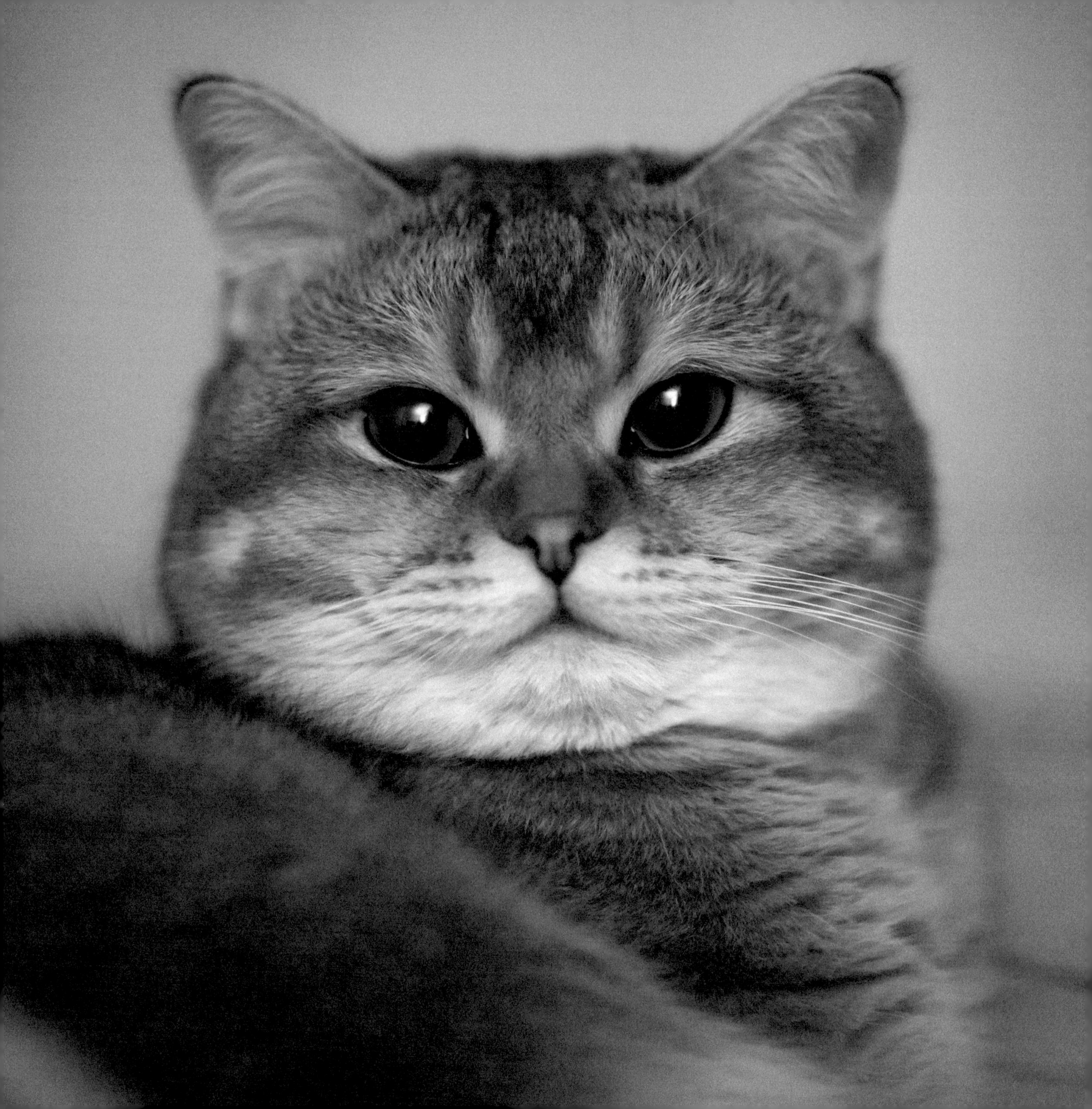

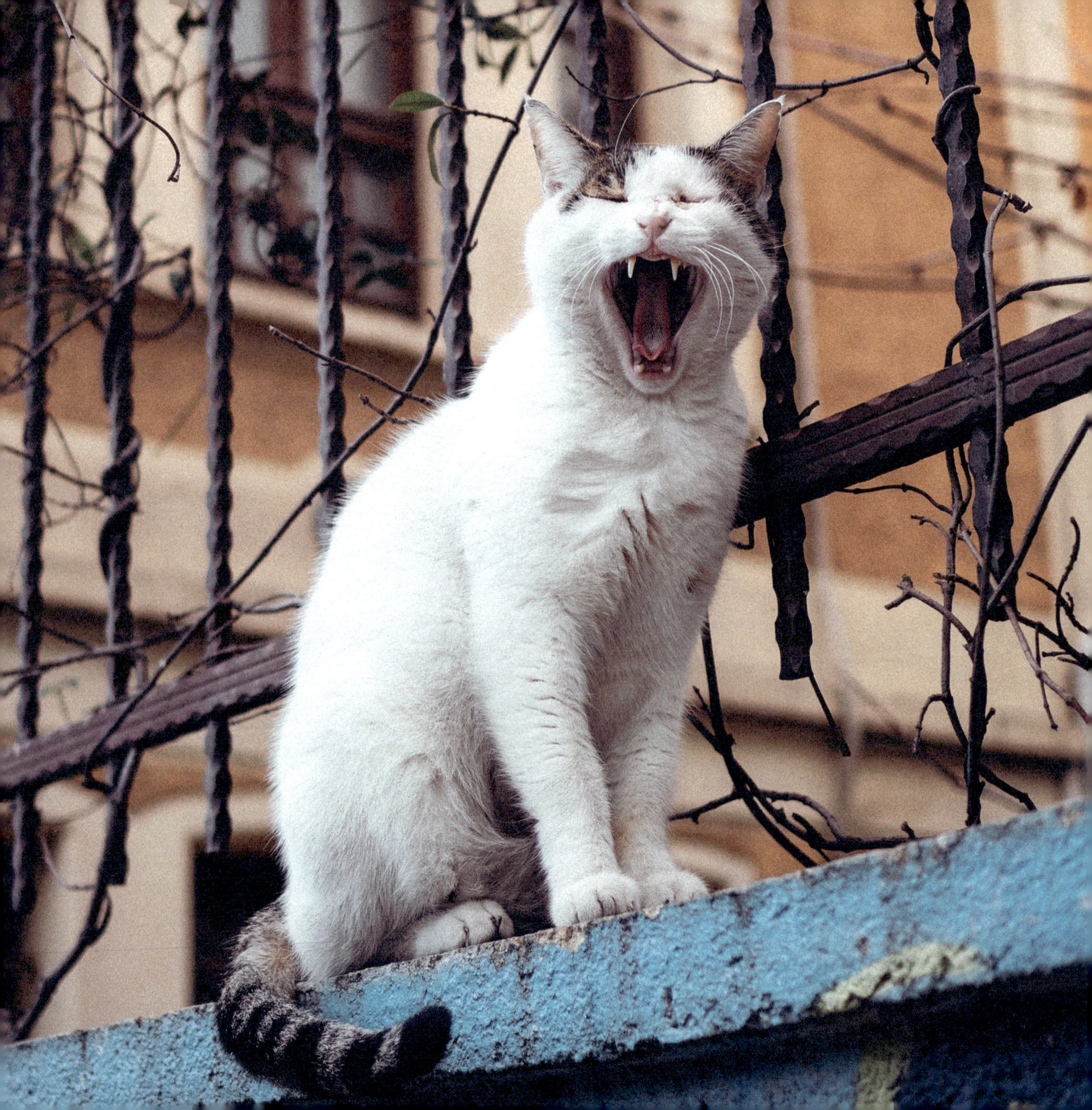

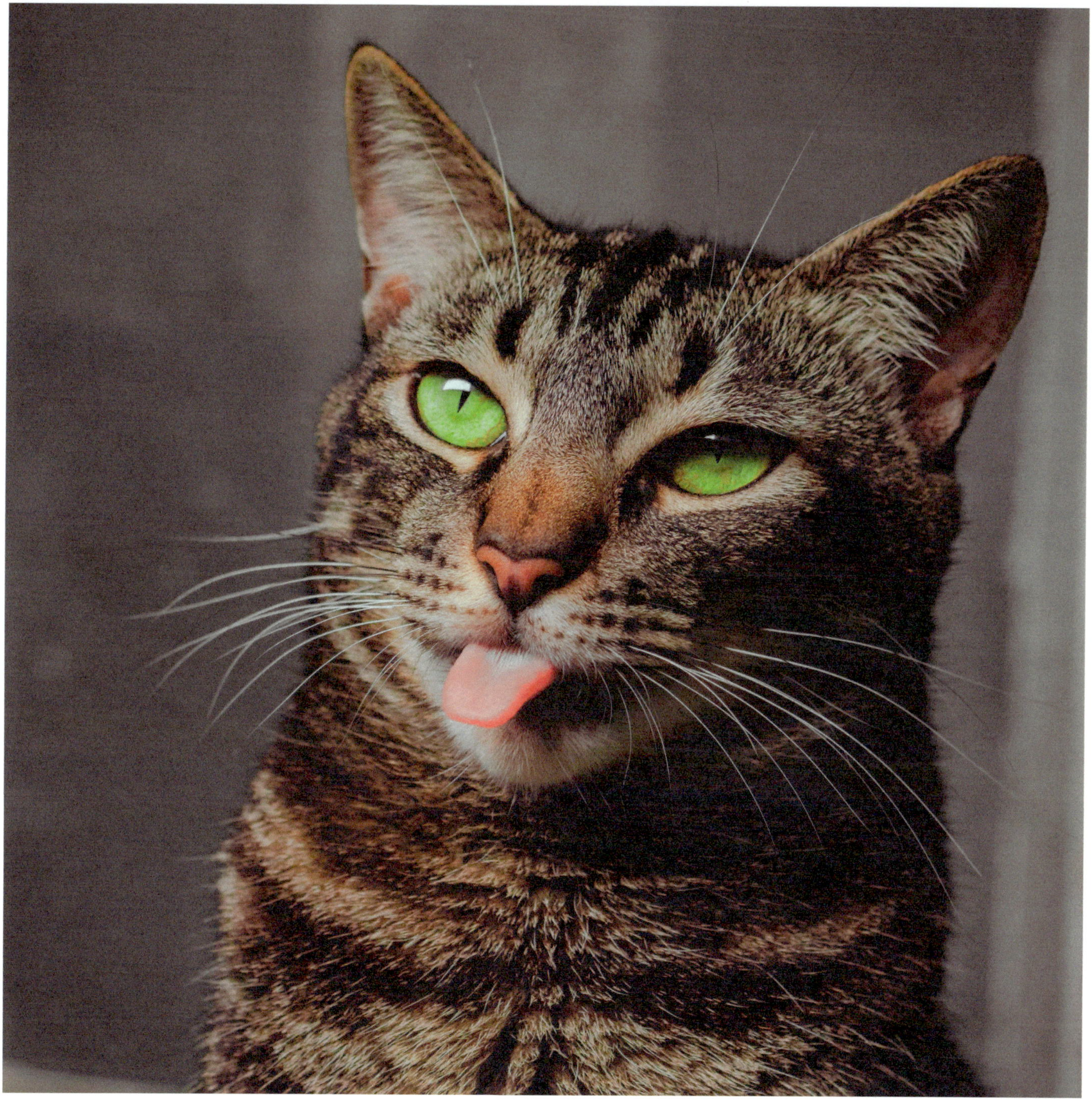

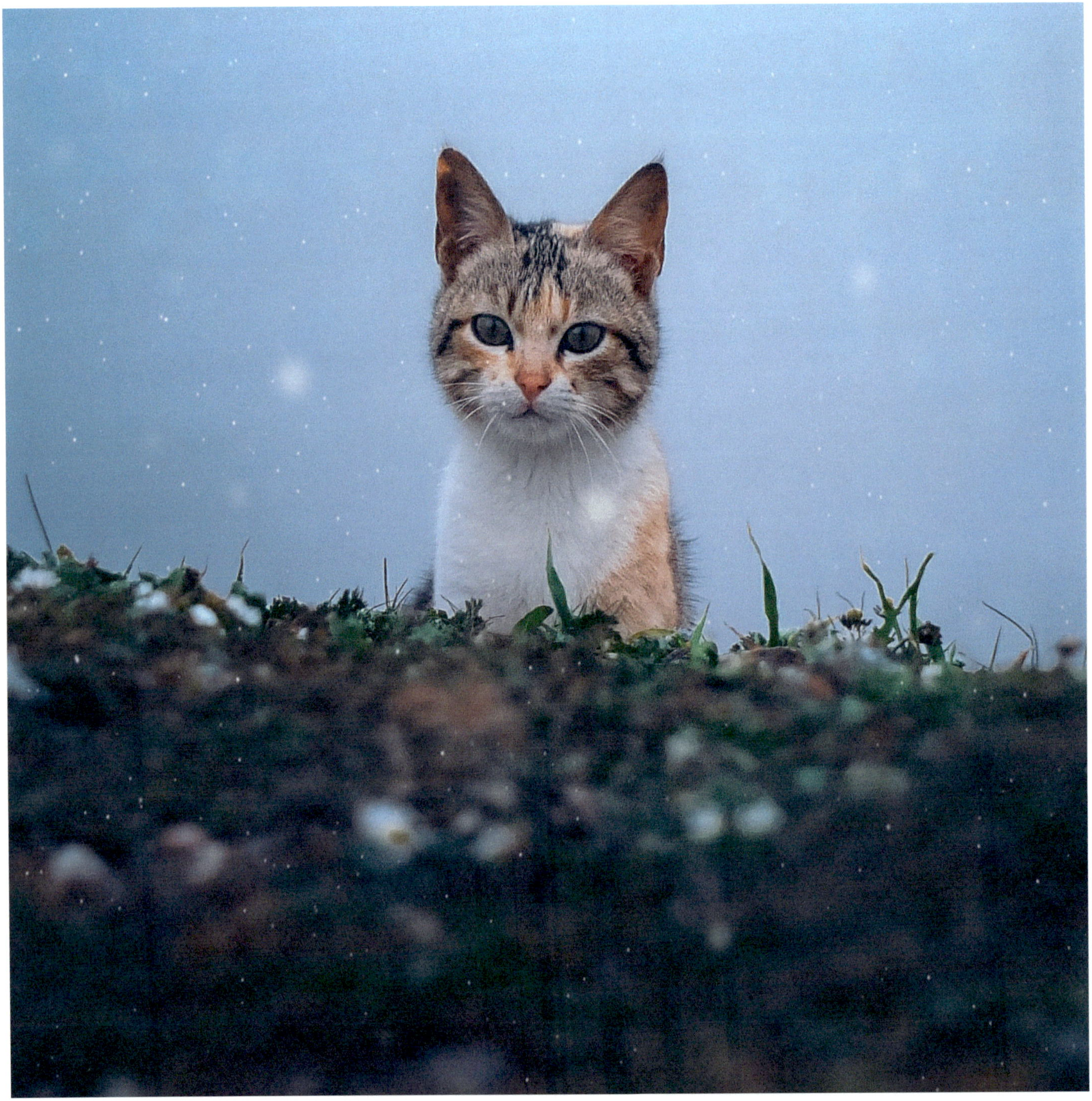

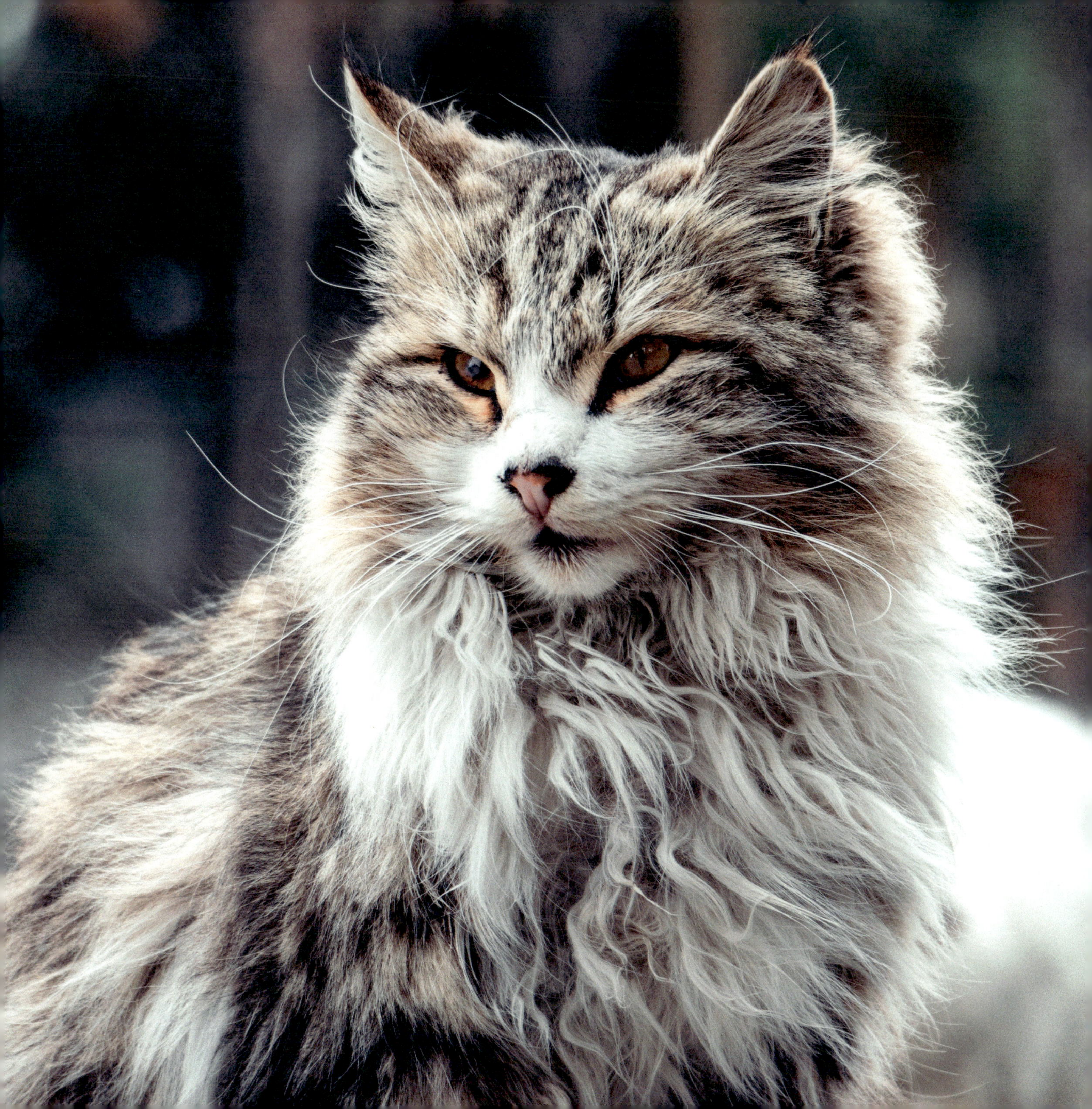

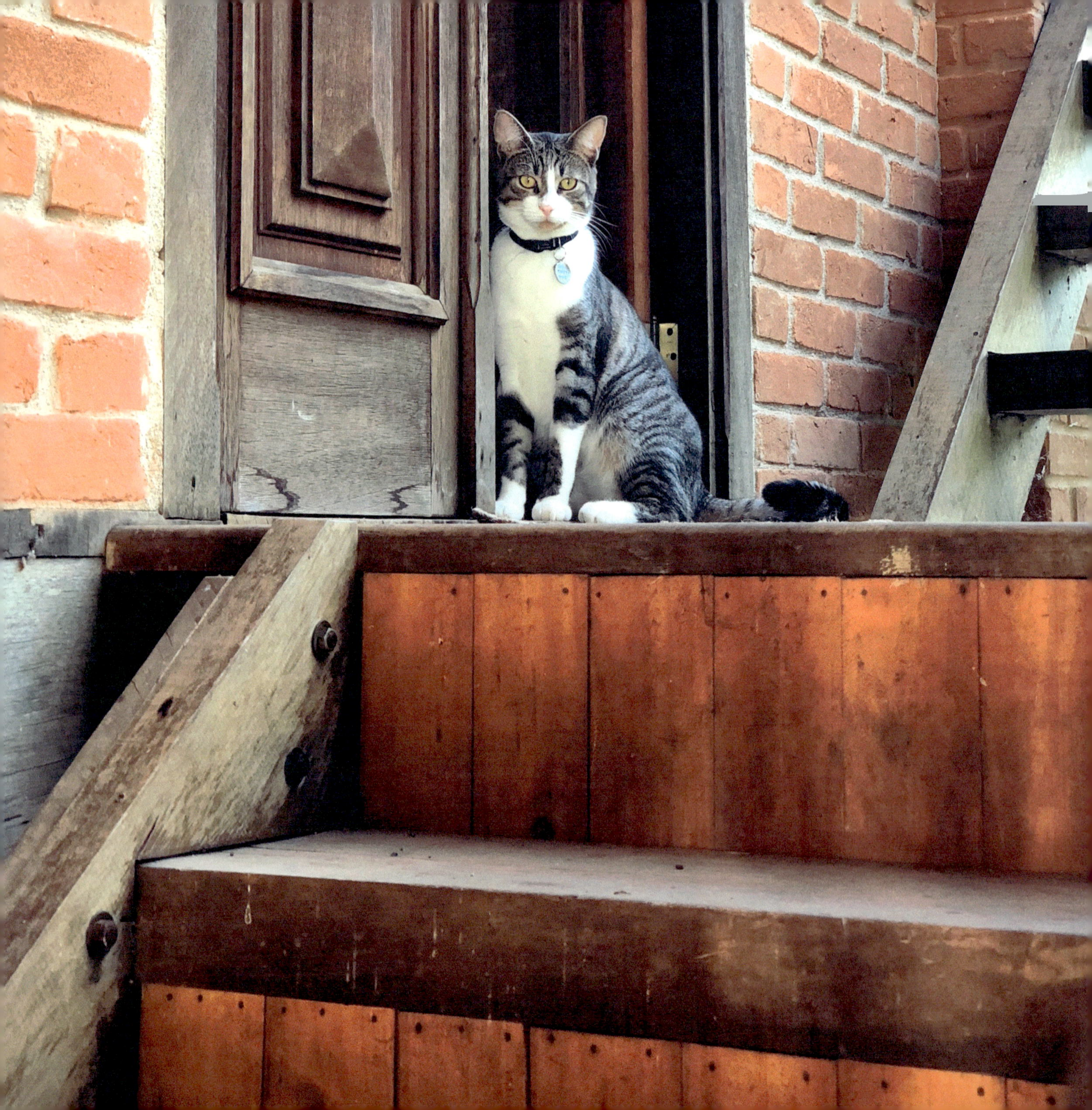

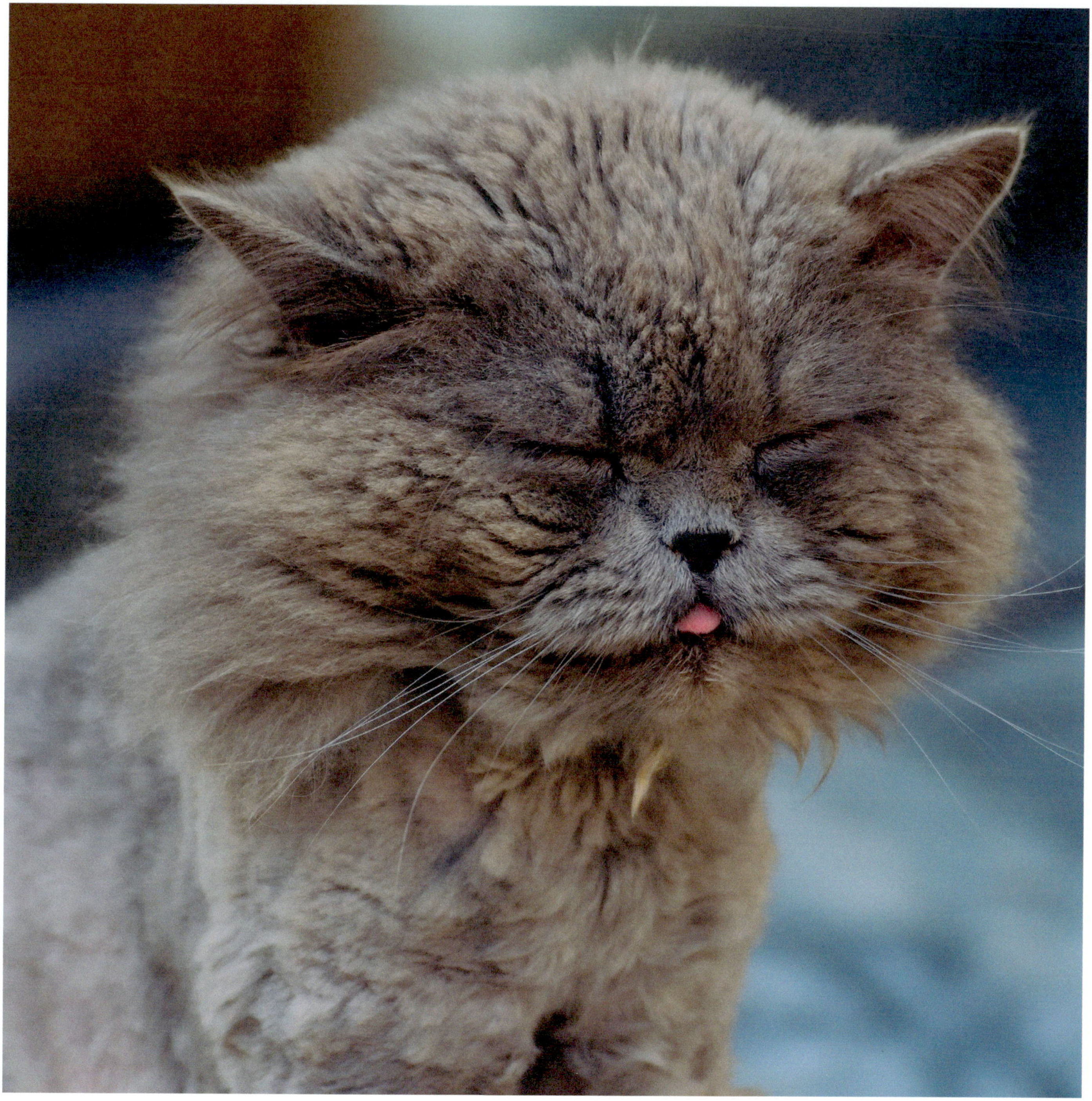

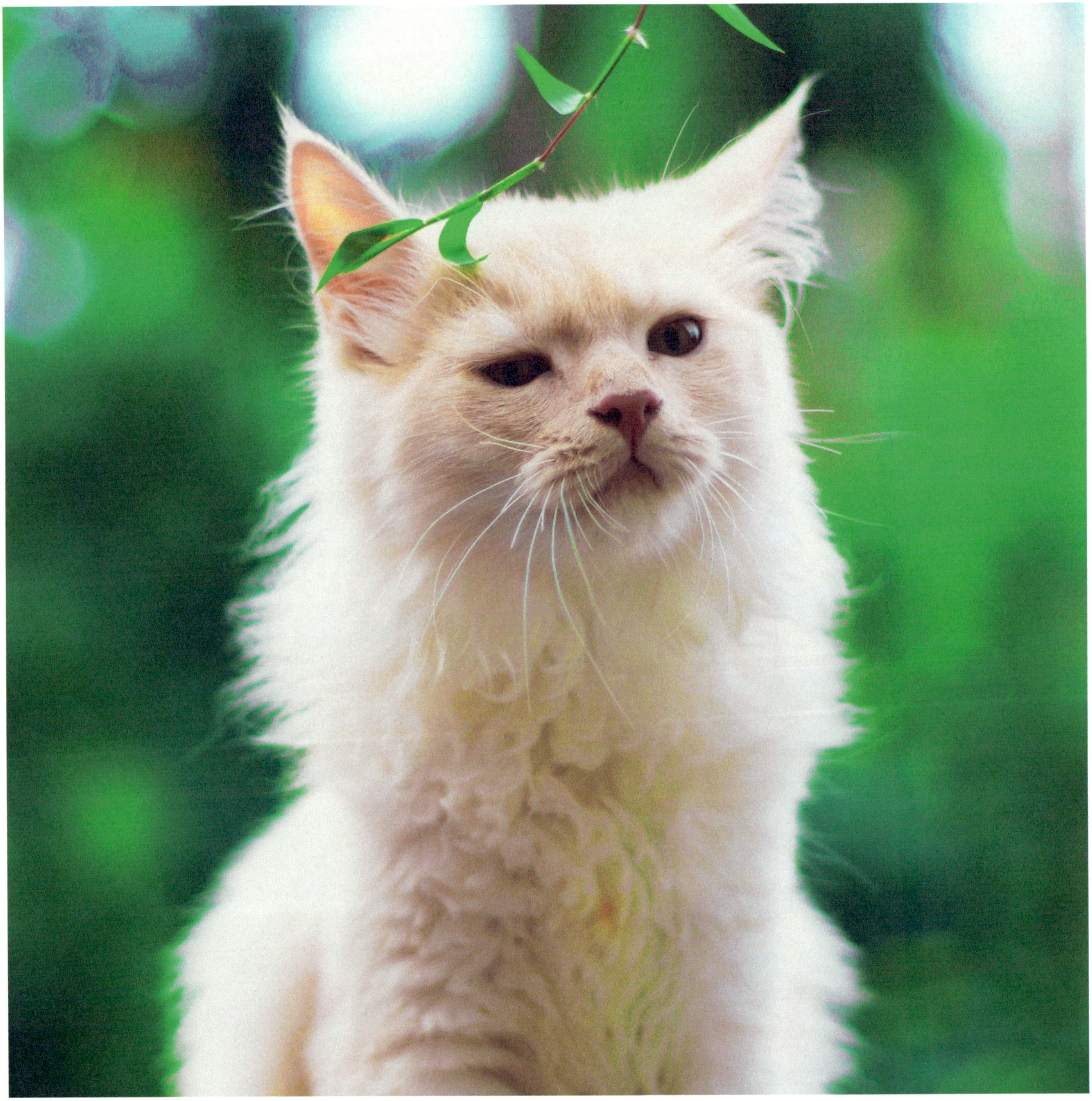

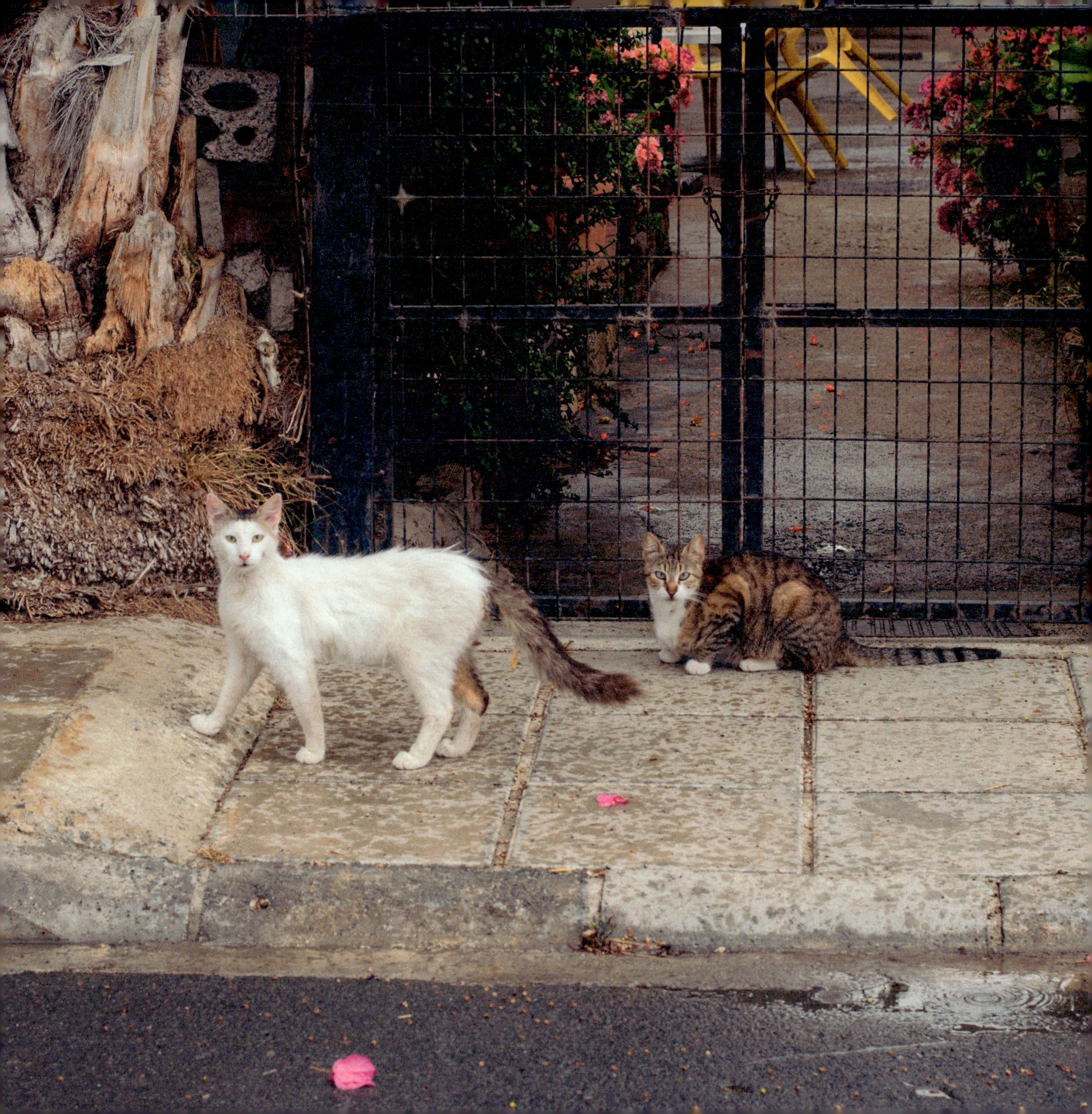

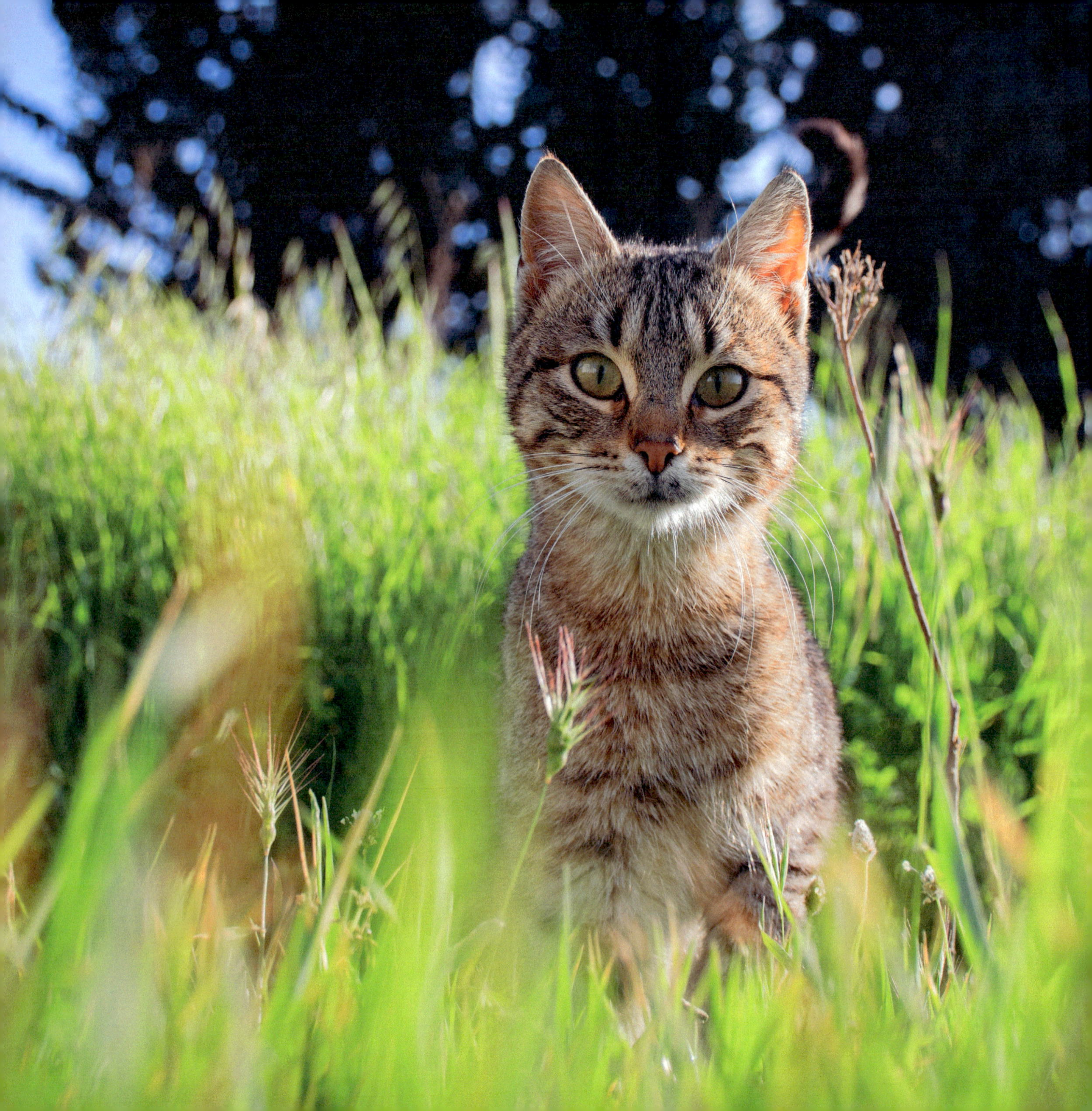

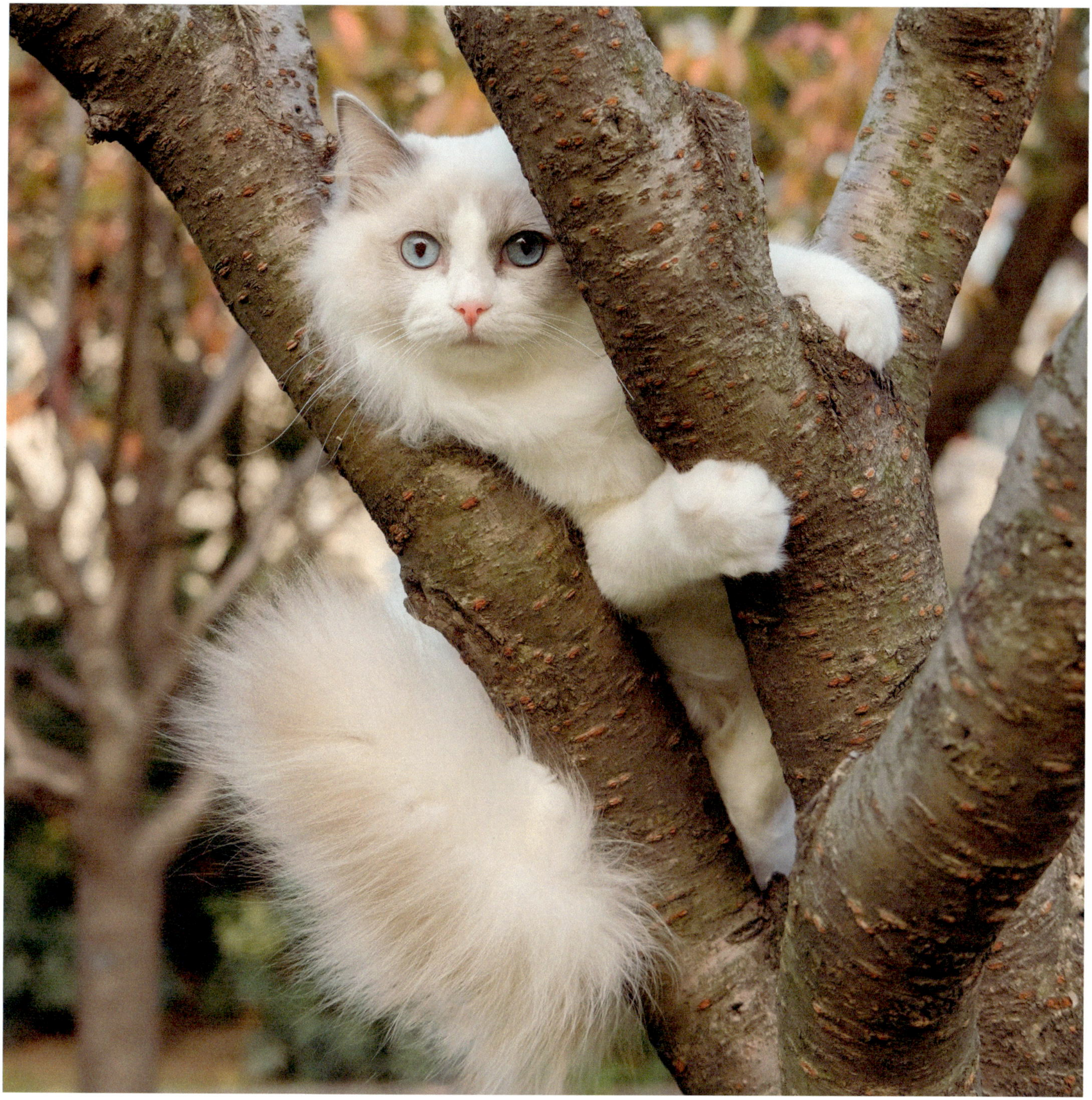

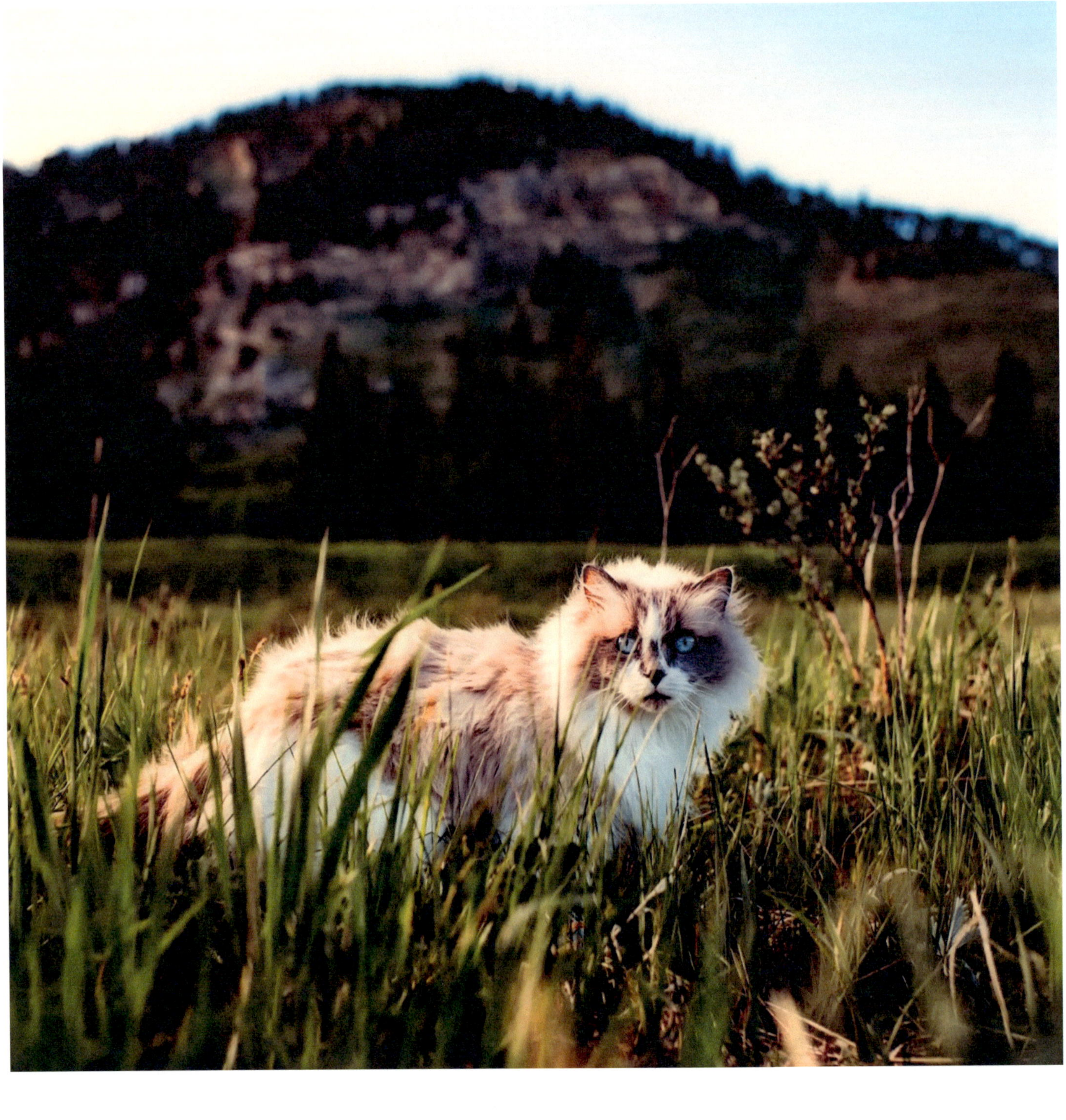

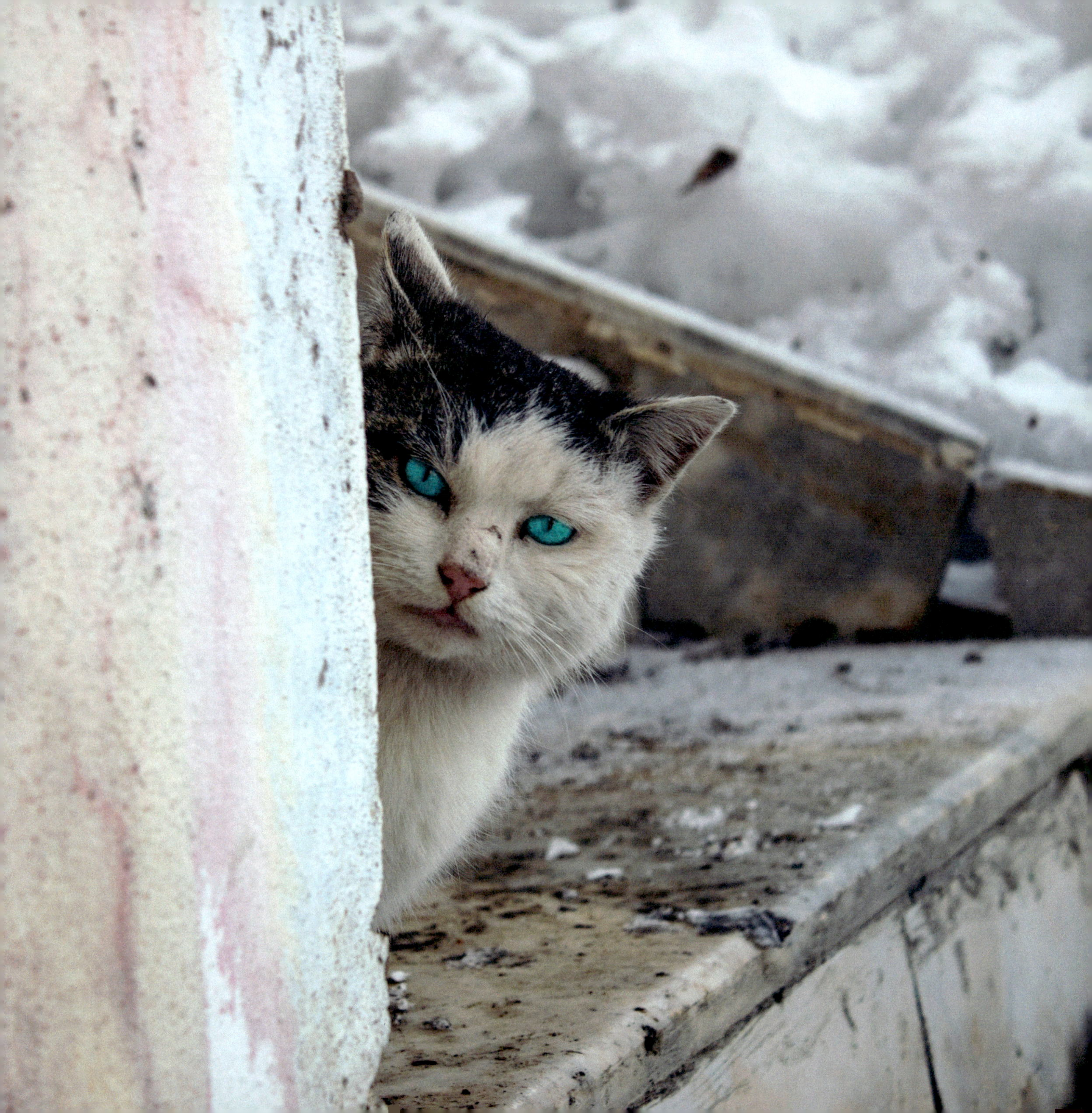

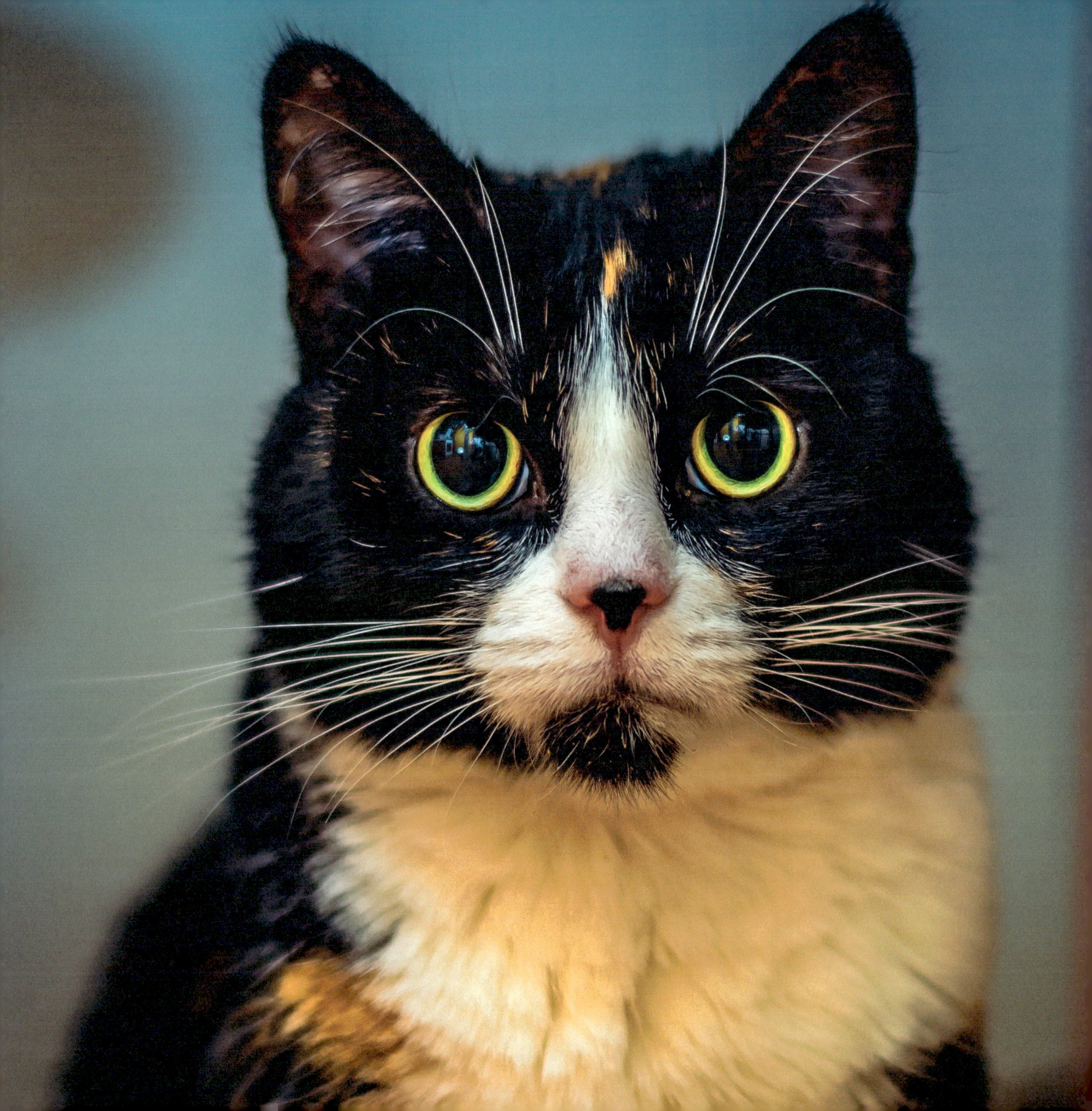

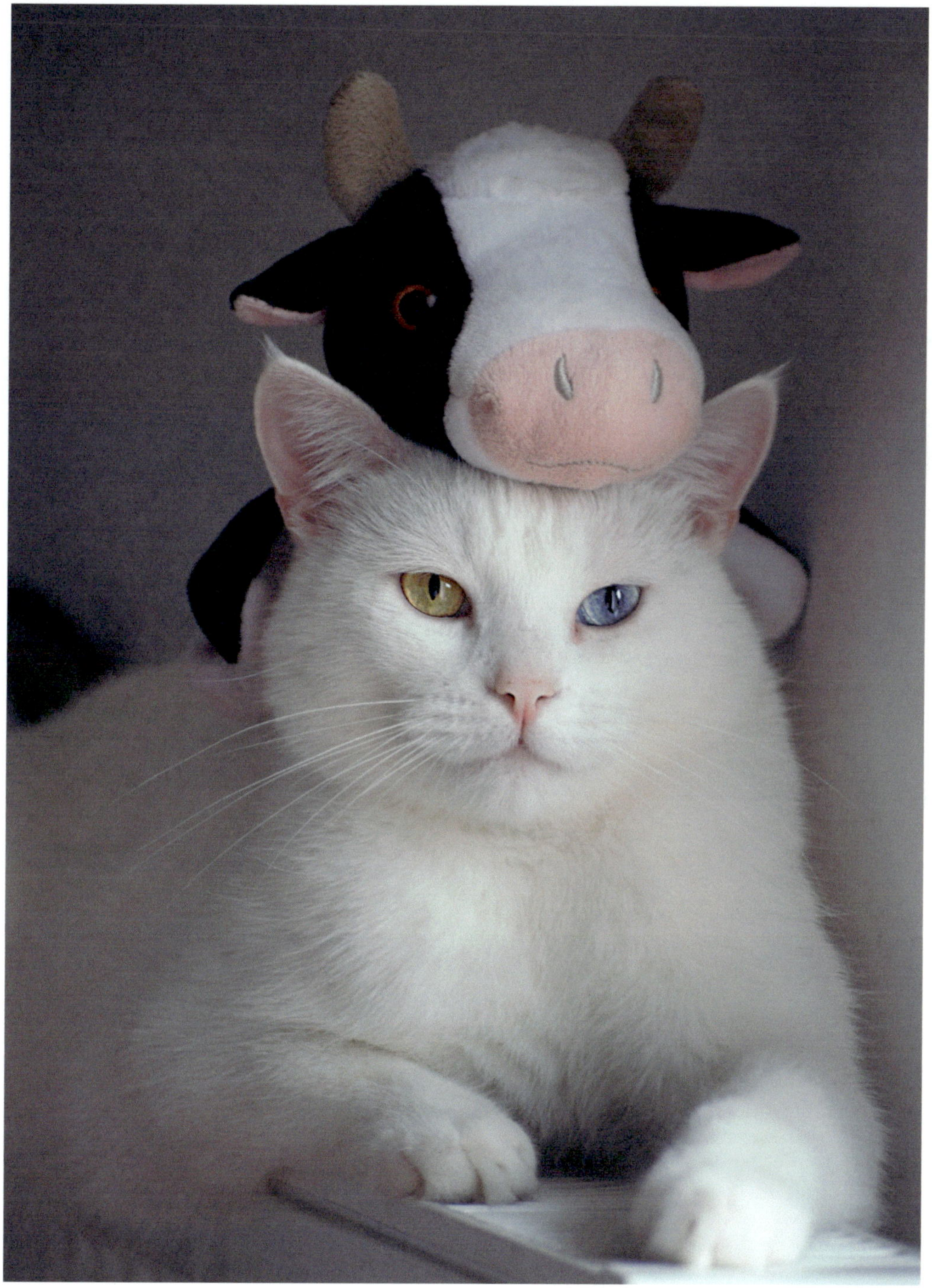

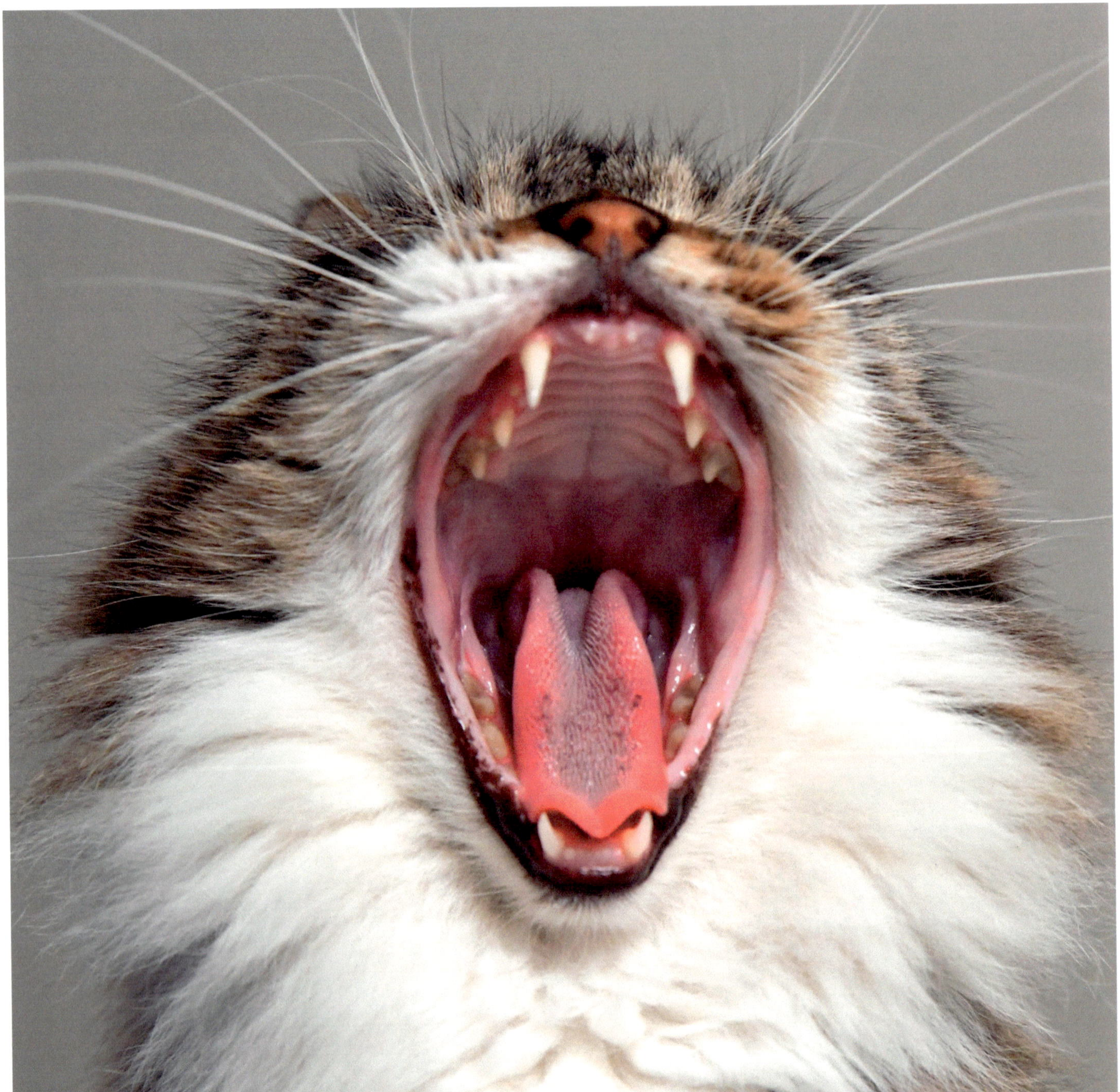

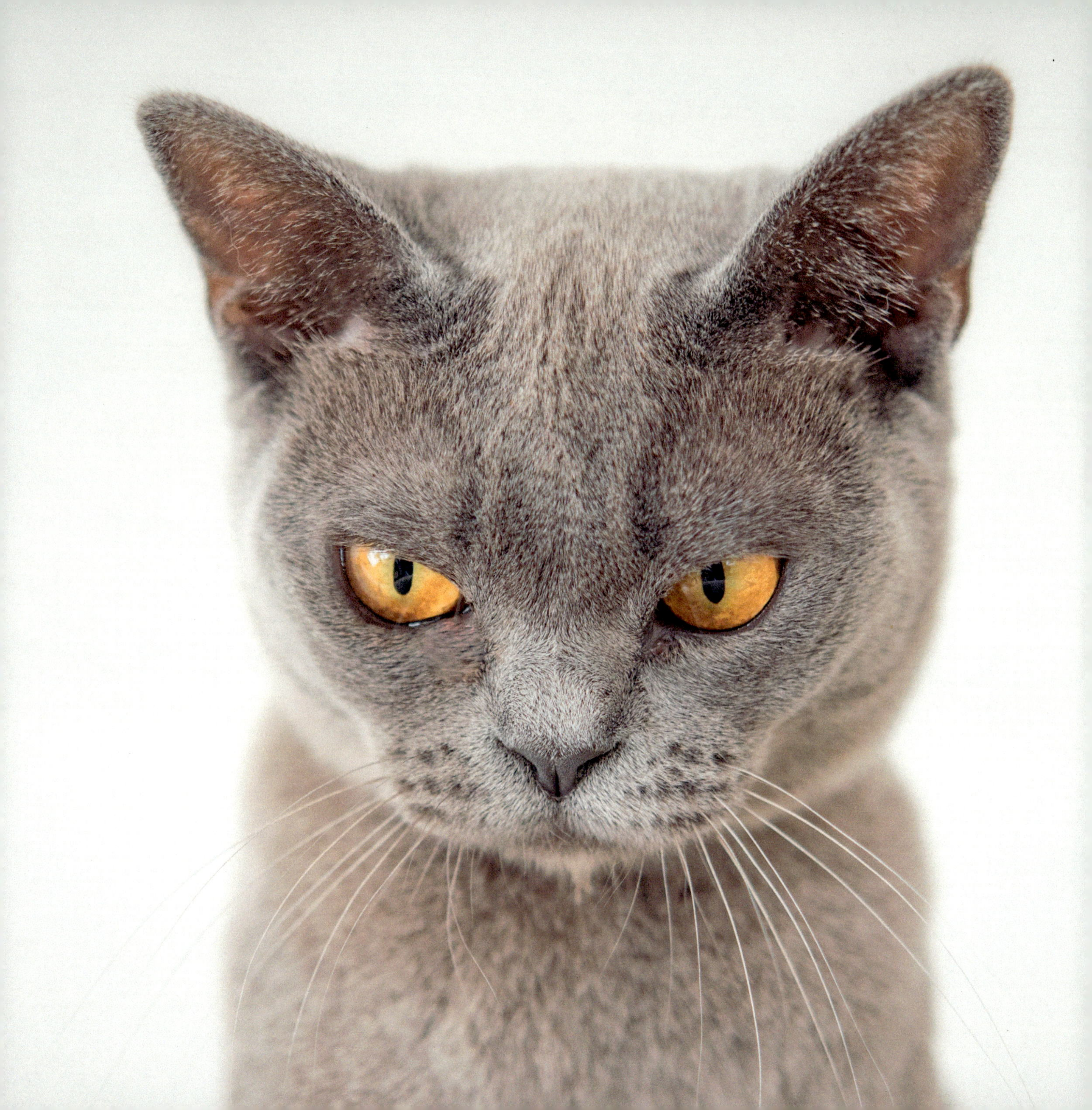

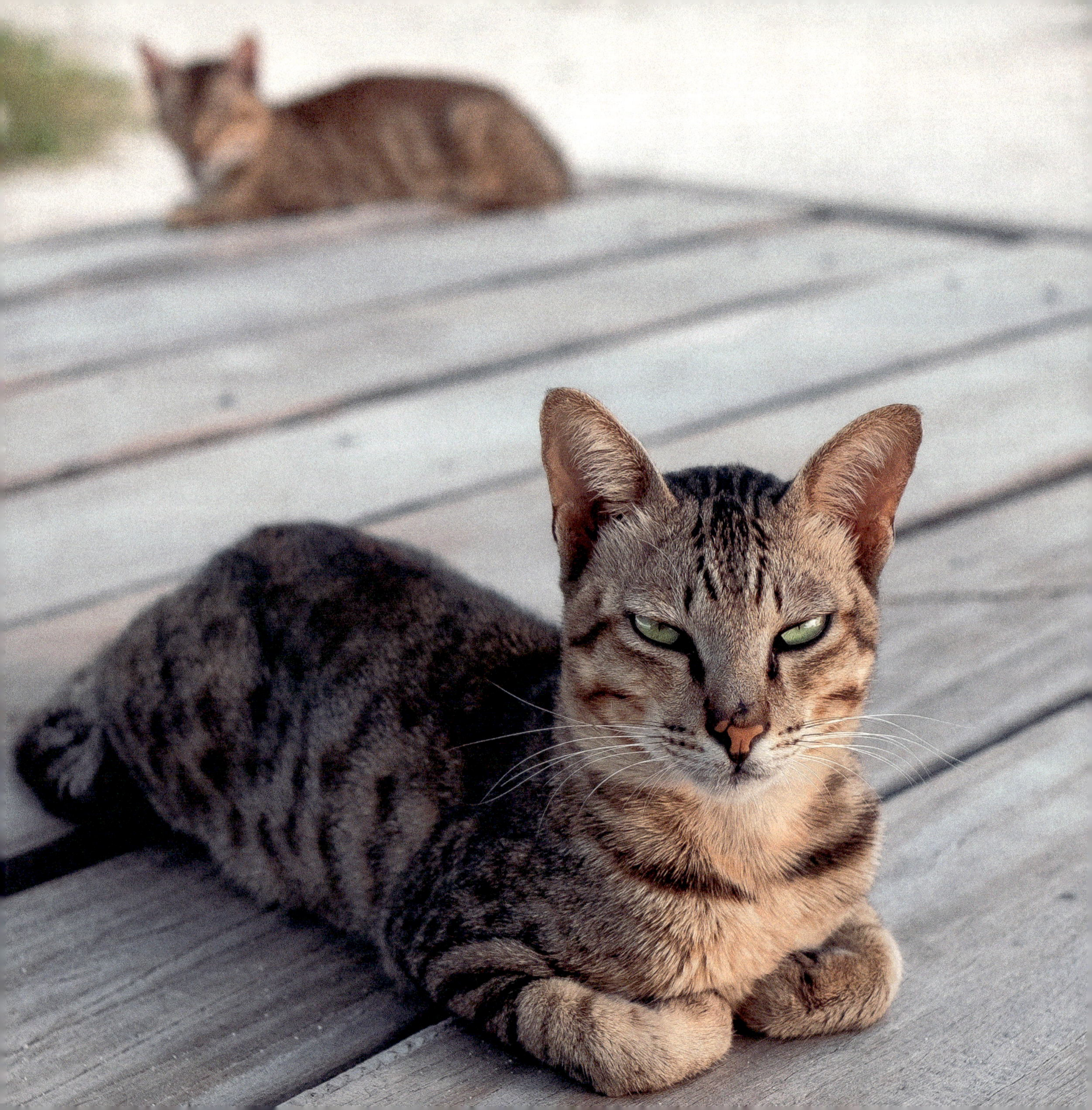

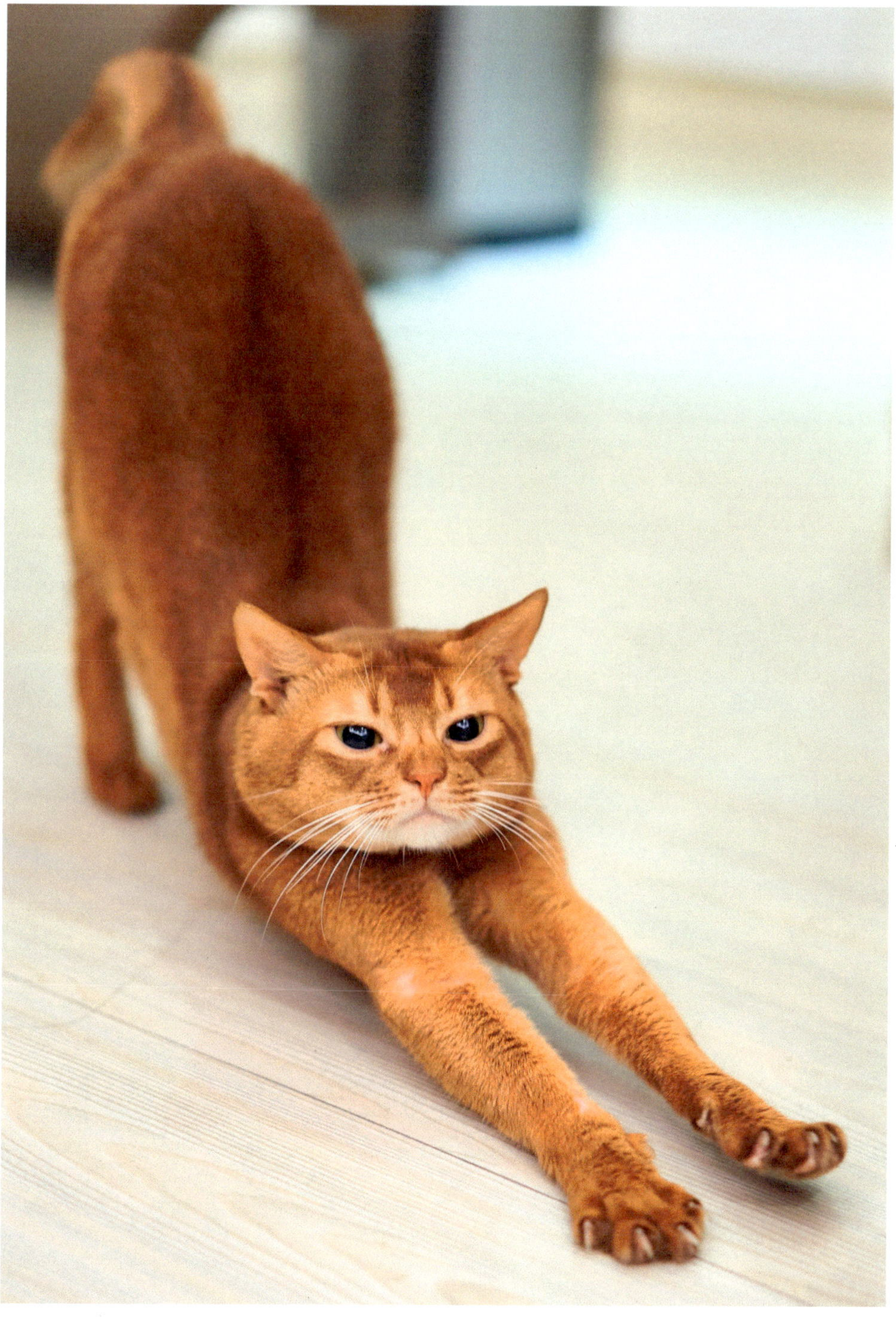

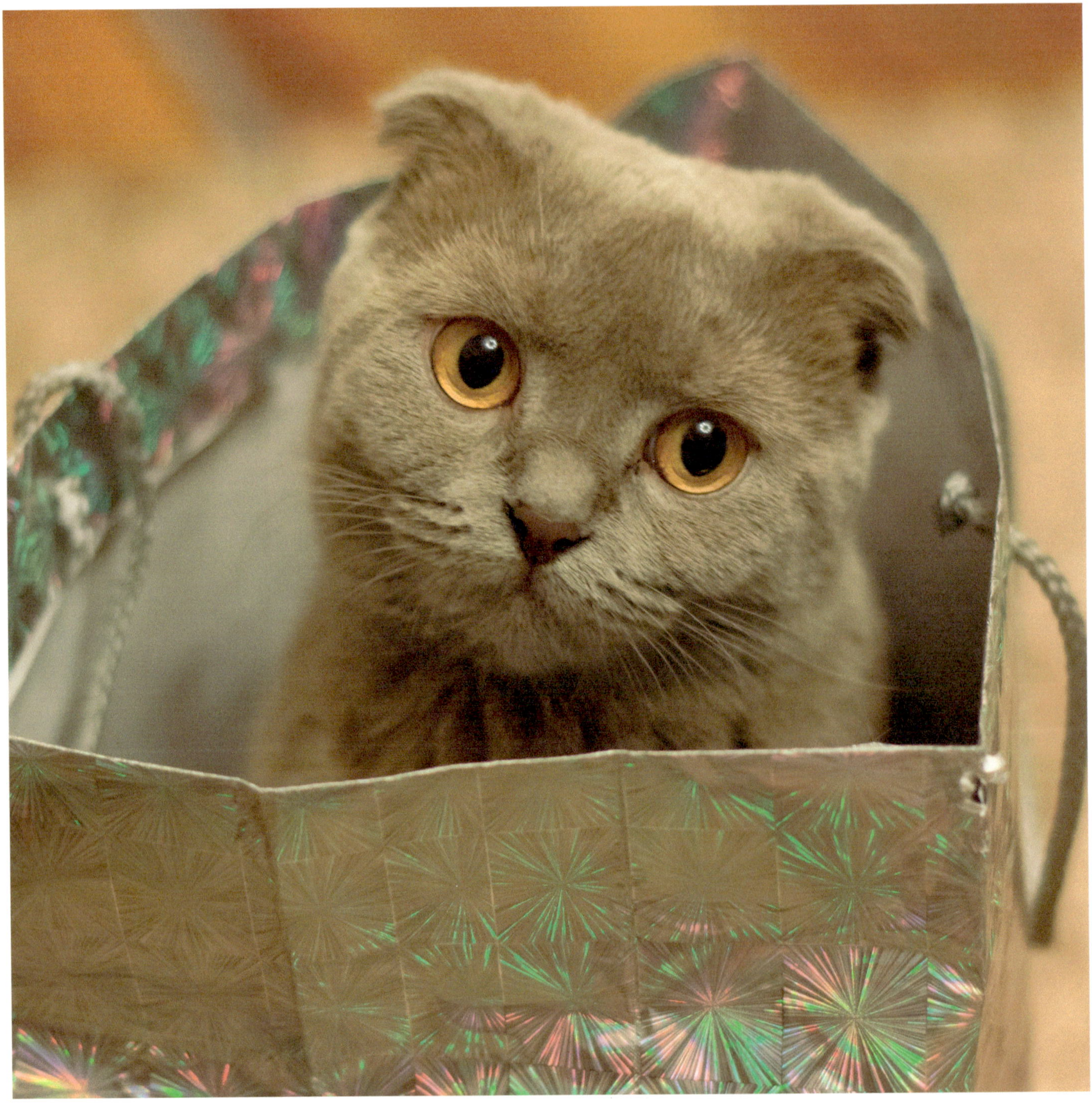

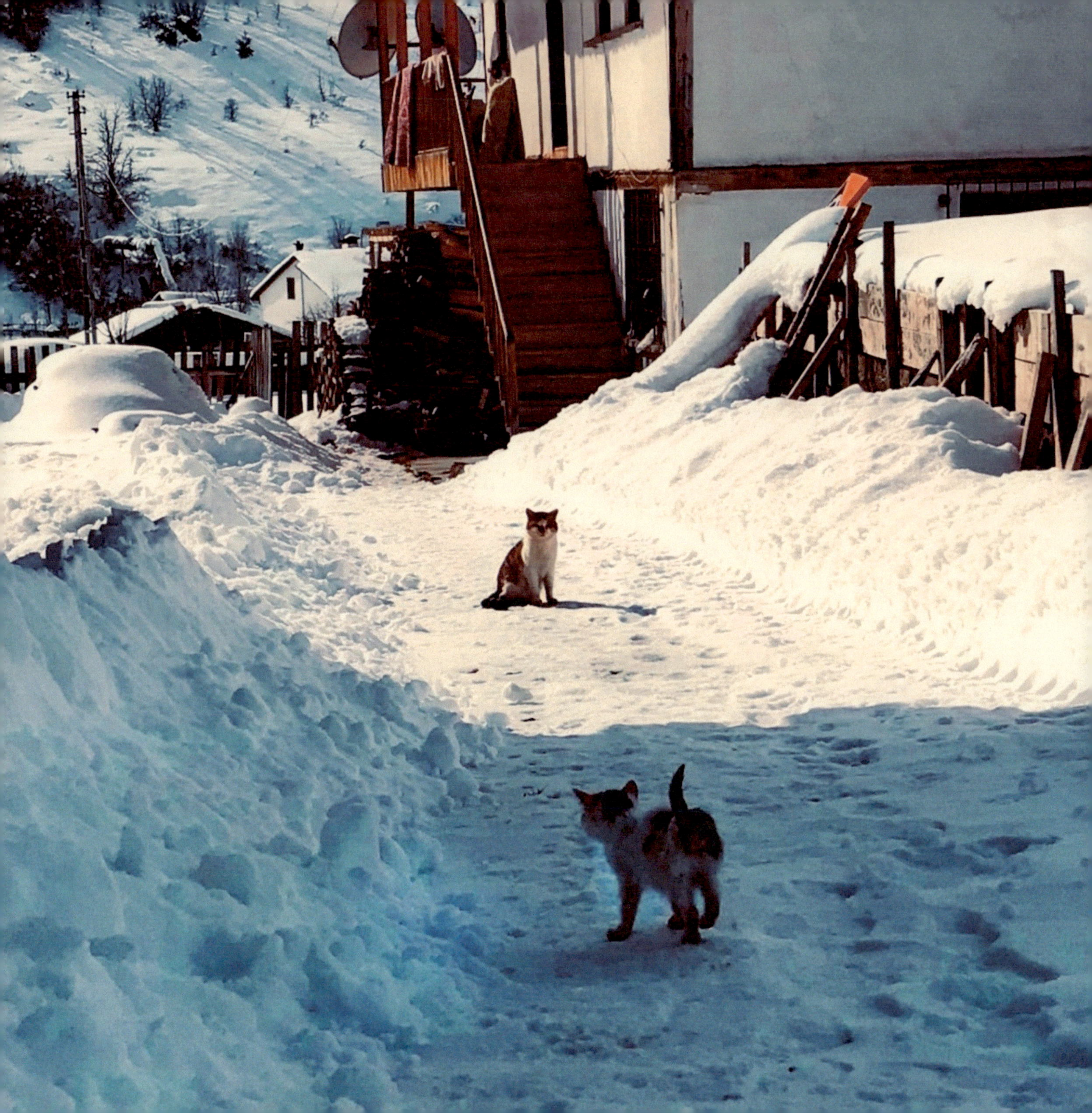

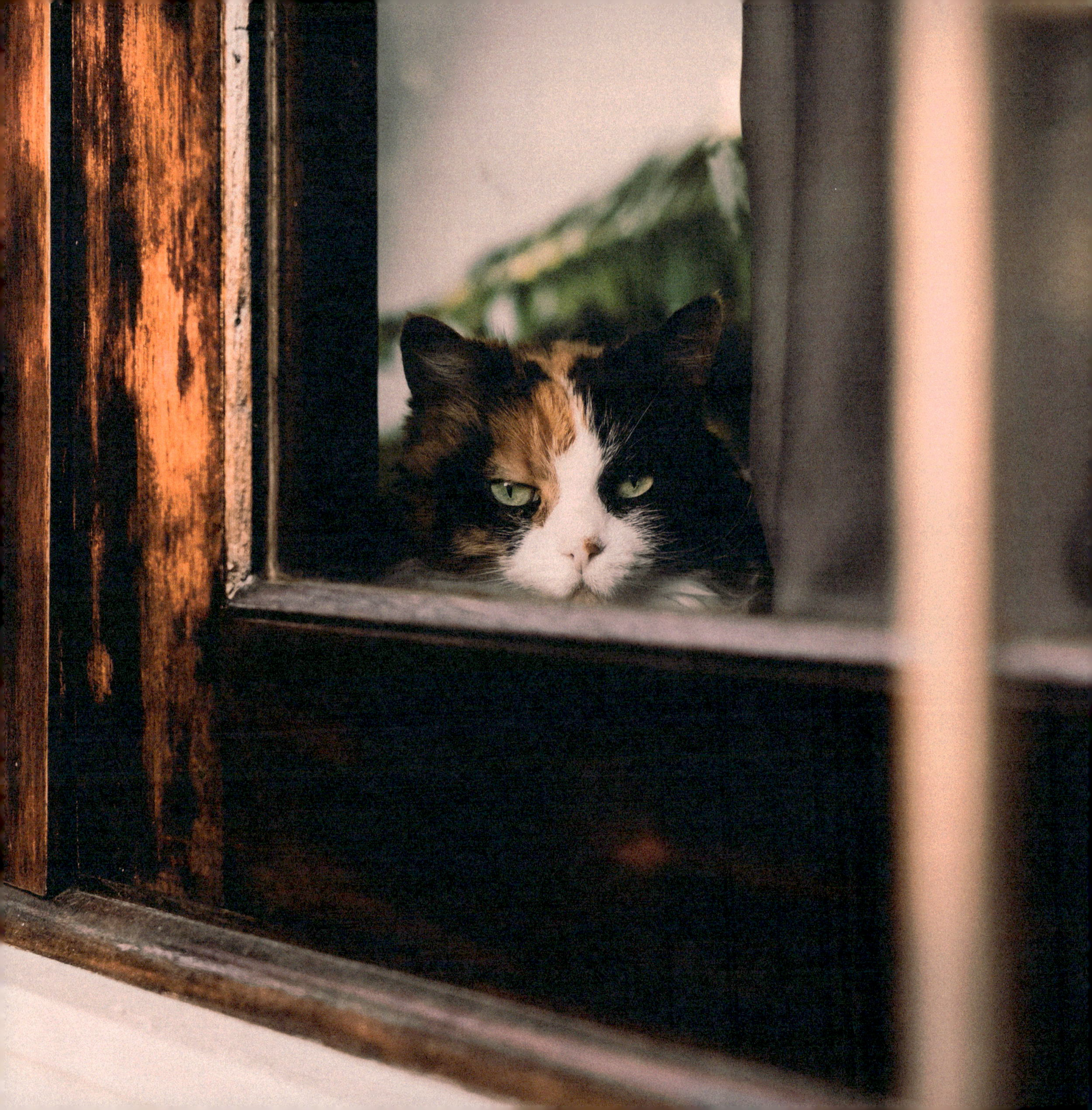

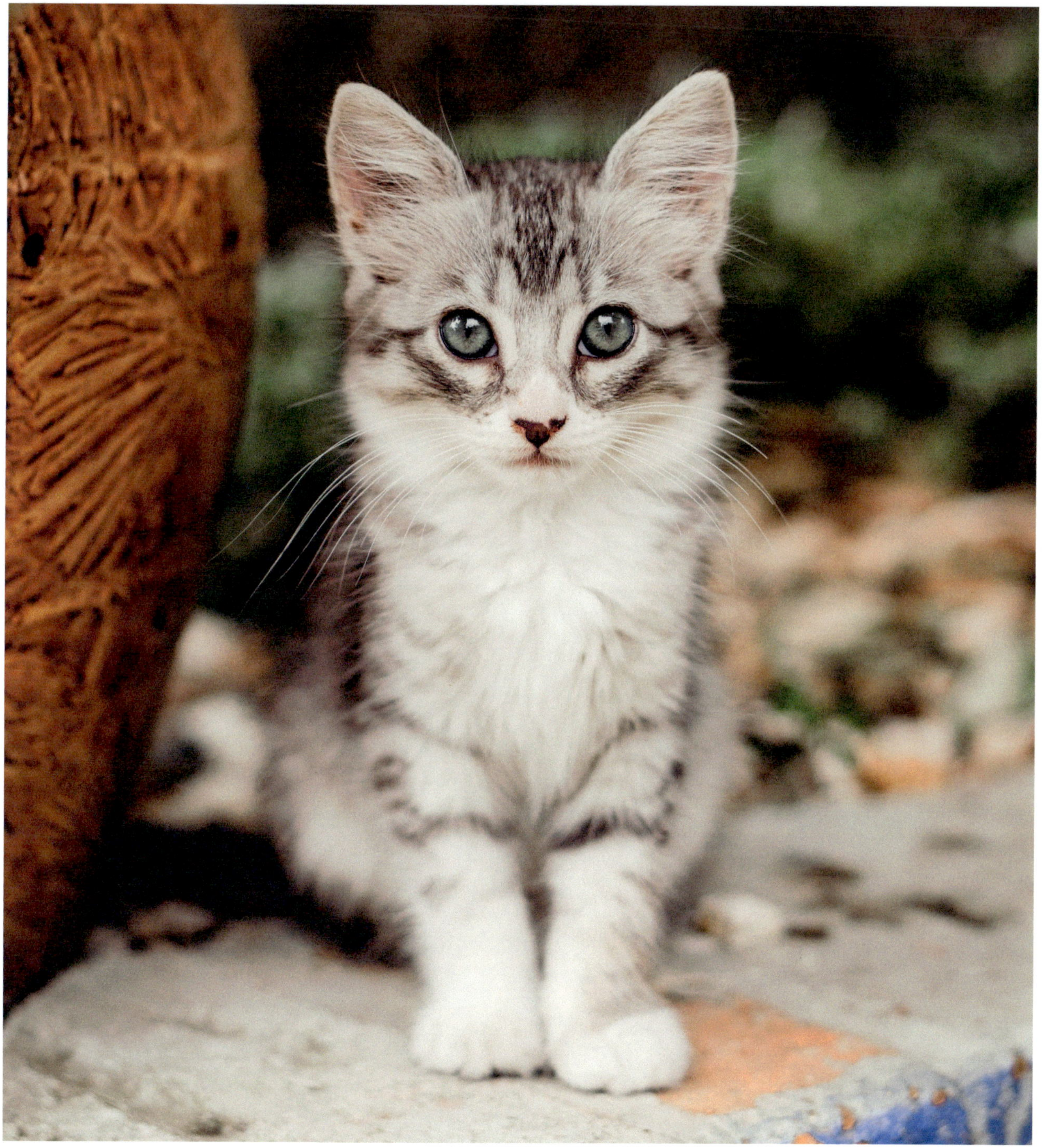

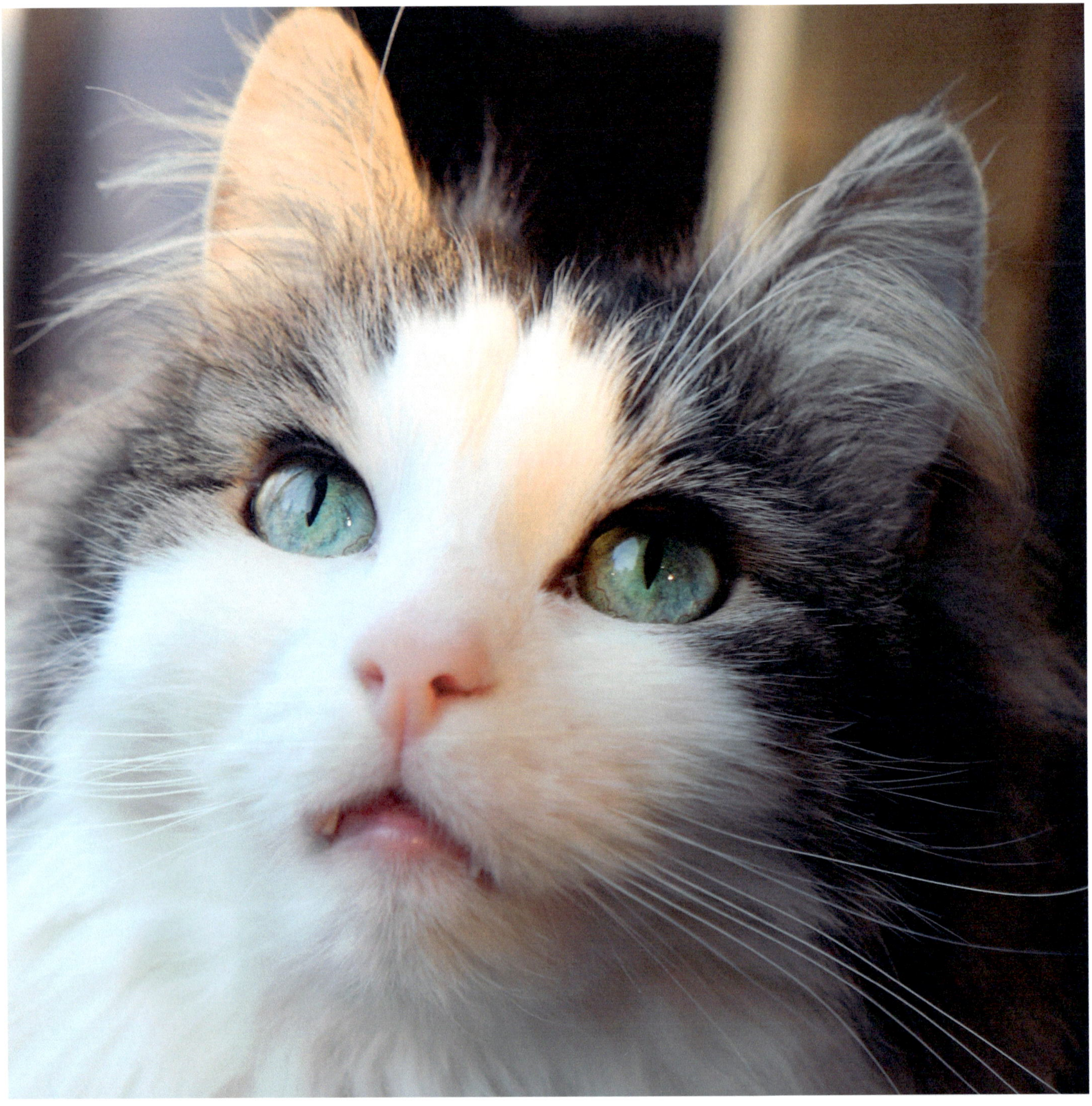

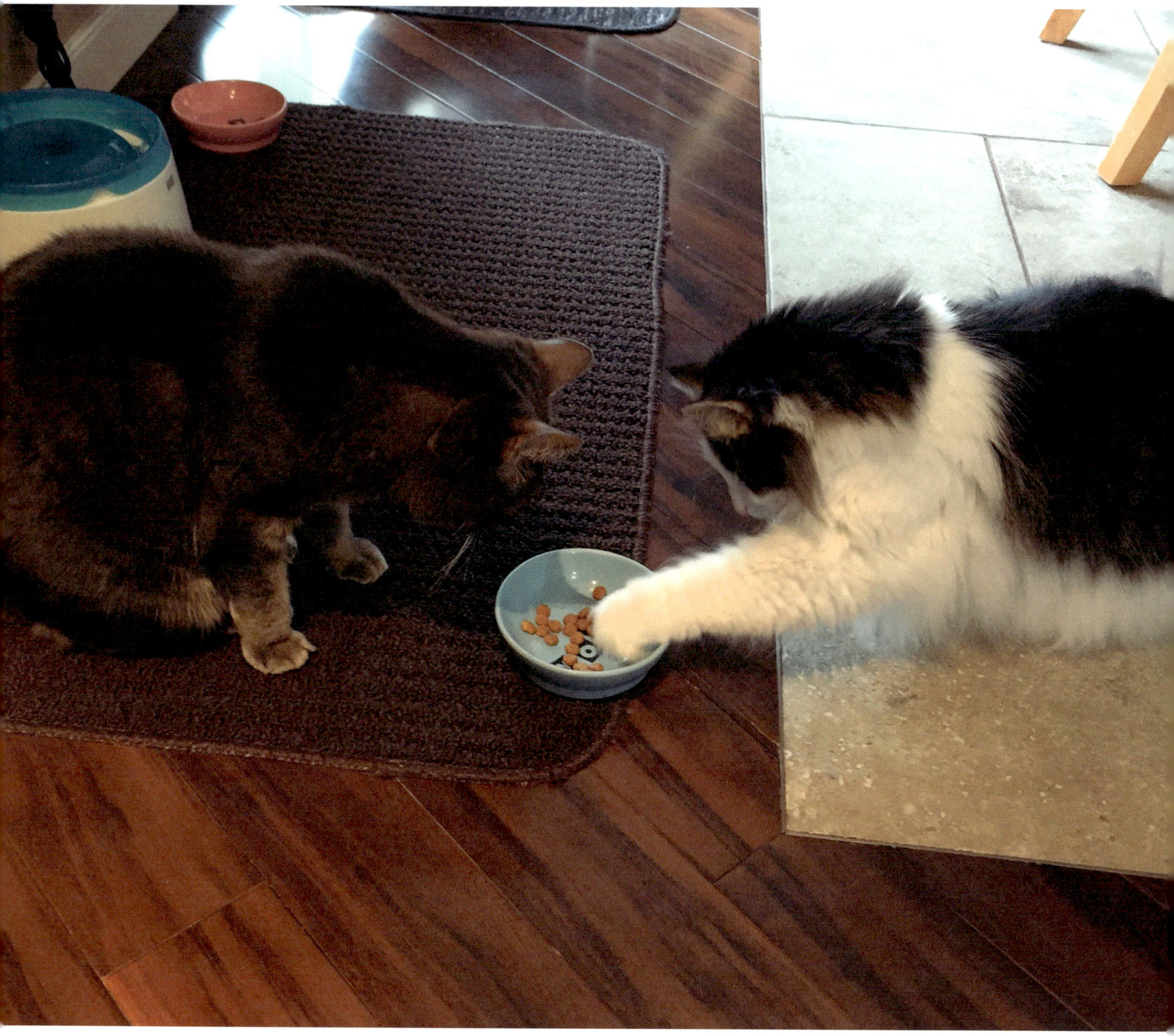

If you enjoyed this book please consider leaving a book review.

Your reviews really help us and others!

Mom And Son Prints

Thank You!

Please send us your feedback
or your book suggestions:
feedback@momandsonprints.com

MomAndSonPrints.com

Made in the USA
Monee, IL
20 December 2025

39677987R00038